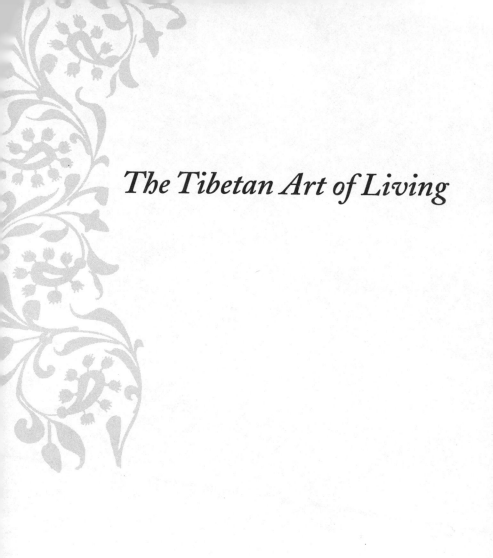

The Tibetan Art of Living

THE

Tibetan Art
OF *Living*

WISE BODY

MIND

LIFE

Christopher Hansard

ATRIA BOOKS

New York London Toronto Sydney Singapore

Dedication

The knowledge in this book is dedicated to the Masters of the Twelve Lores of Bön and the lineages of dMu and Dur. To the Ngagpa of the Nam or "Sky" clan and its lineage, thousand blessings are offered. I dedicate this book to those who read it, may they find lasting happiness.

On a personal note, I dedicate this book to my beautiful wife, Silvia, and my exquisite daughter, Flavia, who supported me with encouragement and love through the process of writing.

Acknowledgments

I would like to acknowledge the valuable support of the following people who made it possible for me to have time to write this book. They are Christopher Walls, Sharon Seager, and Dr. Stephanie Wright.

I would like to thank Fiona Harrold for making introductions and a most wonderful, enthusiastic, and genuine publisher, Rowena Webb. I would like to thank Rosemary Trapnell, Briar Silich, and the art director at Hodder, Ian Hughes, for all his care and attention to detail. Also my thanks to Samantha Evans, Katy Follain, and Jamie Hodder-Williams. To everyone else at Hodder whom I have depended upon, thank you. No book is a solo effort.

To my agent, Kay McCauley, I give deep thanks for helping me on the way to becoming a writer, for her friendship and mentorship.

A deeply important acknowledgment must go to Sarah Stacey, both a brilliant writer in her own regard and an amazing editor who went beyond the call of duty to reveal all the essences of this profound subject while still keeping much of my original text in place. This book could not have been done without her. To Sarah I extend my deep-felt thanks and respect for guidance in helping me to learn about writing.

This American edition of *The Tibetan Art of Living* brings a great deal of satisfaction to me personally, and it would not have happened without the foresight and discernment of Judith Curr and the perfectionism and care and friendliness of Kimberly Kanner. Two special ladies, thank you.

CHRISTOPHER HANSARD
JANUARY 2002

Contents

The Creation of the Universe

According to this Tibetan myth, all living creatures were created seeking harmony and union.

Before time began, before there was Light, there was darkness and all that was, was sustained within a great cosmic egg. Slowly this egg began to crack open. Light, Time, and Space spilled out, becoming the universes, planets, stars, and suns.

From out of the cosmic dust came the Sun and the Moon. The Sun and the Moon traveled through the sky as one, until they were torn apart. From this division were formed the first living beings.

In order to remember their creation, they decreed that the Sun and Moon would come together, once in a lifetime, in a total eclipse that would set in motion the moment when the great cosmic egg would open again, and all things would know their origins.

The Sun, a King, and the Moon, his Queen, longed for each other, dreaming of their reunion. Their dreams became the fabric of human minds and people wanted to dream the same dream as the Sun and Moon. And so in the cycle of a lifetime, the King and the Queen of the Sky would reunite, just briefly, in order to be one again and then part, their tears filling the great void of the sky, spreading their light across time and space.

The Sun and Moon by uniting in a total eclipse remind all living creatures that each is not separate from others. That renewal and transformation is the nature of all things. Thus the King and Queen of the Sky will continue to enfold each other, over and over again, until at last they will stay in the power of their embrace, complete and whole again.

The Song of Wisdom

The fire burned slowly, throwing sparks up into the sunset. The aroma of juniper filled the air, a sacred offering to the god-energies of ancient Tibet. The vibrations from the low chanting of my teacher spread out from the top of Mount Pihanga, where I sat with him. They drifted down into the valley below, blending with the mist.

We were in an area of mountains and lakes in the Taupo region of New Zealand's North Island. It had been sacred to the local Maori people for over a thousand years. In the last light, a river snaking out of a lake glistened palely in the dark surrounding forest. Then night came. Stars leaped out of the void, each one fire bright, each one singing in response to the chant.

My teacher was deep in the flow, his face a study of concentration and stillness. I added more juniper berries and branches to the fire. The flames leaped up as if they were jumping into space. The fire seemed to act as a conduit between heaven and earth, purified by juniper, empowered by chanting.

Picking up a small flat drum, Ürgyen, my teacher, slowly began to move his fingers in long-drawn-out circles over the worn skin. The sound of his fingertips whispered, sussurated. Suddenly a roar burst from the drum, hung in the air, then fell back again, becoming a drone under the words of the chant. A sudden wind blew around us, a continuous stream of magically invoked air. The drum and the wind sounded as one, flowing from the hill out into the wider world.

The hilltop became the only hilltop in the world.
The darkness below was a deep sea of energy.
The energy common to everything that lives and feels.
My mind journeyed into that dark sea, borne by the words of
*   the chant.*
Words from the ancient times of Tibet—of power and blessing,
*   of rebirth and creation.*
Words that free the mind.
Words that destroy ignorance and cast out fear.
Words of healing for every living thing that hears them.

That night I heard the songs of the earth and the elements. The words talked of what we are made of, where we came from, and where we are going. Of how things are. They were songs of wisdom, a wisdom that lies at the foundation of all humanity.

All living things can hear that wisdom. They knew the song my teacher was singing that night. They knew it because they were the words and the wisdom. We know the song, too. Because we are the words. We are the wisdom.

That night, I began to understand and experience the wisdom, healing, and power of this chant, dedicated to endless compassion and wisdom. According to ancient Tibetan belief, it was first sung by the earliest nonhuman inhabitants of Tibet, known as the Masang, who existed well before the dawn of human beings.

The chant was a profound step in my training as a physician of Tibetan Dur Bön medicine. After twenty-three years, spiritual and medical teachings were finally merging into one. As he chanted, my teacher was passing on a spiritual empowerment. The energy released in the process transformed and expanded my psyche, mind, and body. My attachments to my imperfections, prejudices, and obstructions began to dissipate.

The slow droning of the drum reached into every part of me, reorganizing the way I was made, making inner space for consciousness, making room for my humanity to grow, creating spiritual bonds with everything I had learned from my teacher since childhood.

This would be the last year of my teacher's life. He brought many important lessons for me, and I remembered when we first met in New Zealand in 1961. I was on a beach at Rona Bay, Wellington. I was four years old, out for a day by the sea with my parents.

The tide was slowly receding and the sea fell in long gentle waves along the gray-brown sand. There were people in the shallow water gathering small shellfish to cook for their evening meal. Seagulls wheeled and hung expectantly in the wind as I walked along the beach toward the faded, weather-beaten pier.

All that day I'd felt something important was going to happen, something I already knew but did not have the language to express. My parents called me to leave, to go home. But inside me, I knew I could not go yet.

"I have to stay here."

"Come on, it's time to go."

"No, I have to stay."

"Why?"

I didn't know what to say. All my words and thoughts were jumbled. I trudged toward my parents. Then, as we climbed up the beach to the gravel road, I saw my teacher standing there, waiting. A rainbow appeared and he laughed.

Ürgyen Nam Chuk introduced himself to my parents. He explained that he represented a Tibetan spiritual and medical tradition that, among other tools, used a profound system of astrology. This had suggested that I might be a candidate for education in the Tibetan Bön spiritual and medical tradition.

My parents weren't impressed at first. But as they got to know Ürgyen and understood that he was not looking for handouts of any kind, they felt more at ease. They began to understand how important it was for me, and allowed me to go through the next stage, which was a series of tests and spiritual questions to determine whether the astrological process was correct.

My parents were aware of the Tibetan tradition of incarnating spiritual teachers, but Ürgyen explained that he did not regard me as one of these, but as someone who, with training, had the potential to develop rare and special abilities related to medicine, healing, and spirituality in the Bön tradition. I was not regarded as perfect or special and would not be encouraged to think otherwise.

MY TEACHER

Ürgyen Nam Chuk was well known as a Bön Ngagpa, a married man of high spiritual caliber. The Ngagpa tradition is found in most of the Tibetan spiritual legacies from the four Buddhist schools of thought and all the Bön traditions. They are instantly identifiable by their hair, which is worn long and uncut, either in a ponytail or in dreadlocks.

Ngagpas have always been regarded as the spiritual geniuses of Tibet, wild, unpredictable, and incredible. My teacher was like this. Thus, as I grew older I had to be observant and aware in order to avoid practical jokes, booby traps, and the general mayhem that was subtly intertwined with the long hours of discipline, study, and hard work.

Traditionally, Ngagpas perform birth rituals, weddings, funerals, and divinations. They also perform a wide range of other rituals, simple and complicated, for the protection and benefit of their communities. All Ngagpas are credited with having power over and with the forces of nature. The weather and the harvest come under their aegis, for example, as do the dispensation of justice and, sometimes, warfare. Some are also experts in martial arts, some are master physicians, and others are great spiritual masters. Ürgyen was one of the few who had developed all of these qualities.

He came from the Nam clan, which had originally entered Tibet from Lake Baikal in Siberia well over eight hundred years ago. They were famous for their medical skills, spiritual teachings, and psychic powers. Although the Nam were partly nomadic, they intermarried with local people and finally settled permanently in the Tibetan province of Amdo. Another group based themselves in Nangchen Gar, a small self-ruling kingdom within Tibet, which became an important spiritual center for the Ngagpa tradition.

The entire clan left Tibet in 1916, almost forty years before China invaded Tibet. An important master within the Nam lineage had prophesied the invasion and—with others—tried in vain to warn the Tibetan authorities. The complete Nam clan moved from Tibet and, under instruction from the head of the clan, split into various units so that each could look after a special part of their culture and set up a trade network.

Some went to Nepal, a few to Leh and the little kingdom of Lo, while others went to Himachal Pradesh, a state in India. Others journeyed to Sikkim, and to another state of India called Arunachal Pradesh, or to Calcutta, Bombay, Varanasi, and Madras. The people who represented the spiritual core of the Nam clan kept themselves secure in remote parts of

Sikkim and the kingdom of Lo. As my teacher grew up, he traveled to all of these places to gain inner knowledge, and he was also involved in managing the wealth of the clan.

Every year, astrological divinations were carried out concerning the spiritual teachings of Bön. Eventually it was decided that for the teachings to continue, suitable people had to be found outside the clan, perhaps even outside the Tibetan community. The divinatory masters built a structure on the ground representing the earth and the astrological influences and, after much study, directed my teacher, then in his late thirties, to search in the Southern Hemisphere for a suitable person. He arrived in New Zealand four years before I was born.

EARLY DAYS

From the age of four, I spent the next twenty-three years of my life learning the spiritual and medical knowledge of ancient Tibet. My family had moved from Wellington to Auckland by then, and I went to a normal Western school and was a typical naughty boy. My teacher followed and I saw him at the beginning and end of each weekday and on weekends.

At eight, my formal Tibetan medical education began, alongside the spiritual disciplines I had been learning since I was four. I also learned the Bön version of the exercise system called Kum Nye, which consists of eight exercises designed to transform the mind and body, clearing obstructions, improving physical strength and health, and preparing the student for higher stages of learning.

WE ARE OUR OWN HEALERS

"To heal someone, you must first know why people suffer," my teacher said. "If, through healing them, you can show them how to stop suffering, you have fulfilled your role as a physician."

I learned that at the heart of all suffering there is a spiritual remedy that comes about from knowing the relationships between karma and suffering. Karma comes from the chaos that exists within all living creatures, all aspects of this world, and the universe at large. Some chaos is good, some indifferent, some bad, but it is the stuff from which happiness and then enlightenment can be made.

By transforming chaos within the mind and body, the physician of Tibetan medicine gives the patient opportunities for healing, happiness, and wisdom. Meditation and the generation of compassion are at the heart of this body of knowledge because, without these resources, the knowledge could easily be used in unskillful ways.

Healing is not taught. It is a continual stream of energy that flows from human consciousness into the natural and man-made world. Through the techniques, observations, and theories of Tibetan medicine, you can learn to connect with this continual stream of healing.

Healing is also an aspect of love, of an expanding compassion that comes from the drive of consciousness to seek itself. In the world, the universe, and within ourselves, consciousness seeks to bring all chaos into balance, so that matter, time, and space will disappear into a continual flow of harmony. Healing is not just making a sick person better; it is making that person more conscious.

Healing is an act of self-knowledge, too. We are our own healers. When we know that we need healing, we activate the healing within us, which awakens knowledge about who we are. This can also be stimulated by the physician responding to a patient's request for help.

As I studied, my self-knowledge matured (at least in my own mind) and my awareness of the immensity of Tibetan medicine increased, year by year. At fourteen, I took the vow that all Tibetan physicians take in my tradition: "I vow to work until I am no longer needed, when illness in all its forms and guises has gone, and all living beings have achieved lasting happiness."

The moon rose high upon a garland of stars, its light spreading faintly across the sky. I could see the river and lake below me. The firelight splashed across my teacher's face, showing his deep state of meditation. Occasionally, shooting stars rushed past.

"Each one is a soul coming back to birth again," he said softly.

I found myself reflecting silently on the strangeness of this experience. Sitting on a sacred mountain in the sacred land of the Maori people, learning Tibetan sacred teachings with the blessings of Maori elders on my teacher. Making sense of it all seemed a challenge.

My teacher knew my mind. "Don't deny your own culture, learn from it as much as you can," he said. "Try to bring a unity between what I have tried to teach you and what is in the West."

His words activated a growing and changing consciousness within me. I felt a blending of energies within me of West and East: Tibet and the Antipodes, Bön and New Zealander— ancient knowledge from the top of the world delivered to a young man in a young country perched at its end.

CHRISTOPHER HANSARD
LONDON, 2001

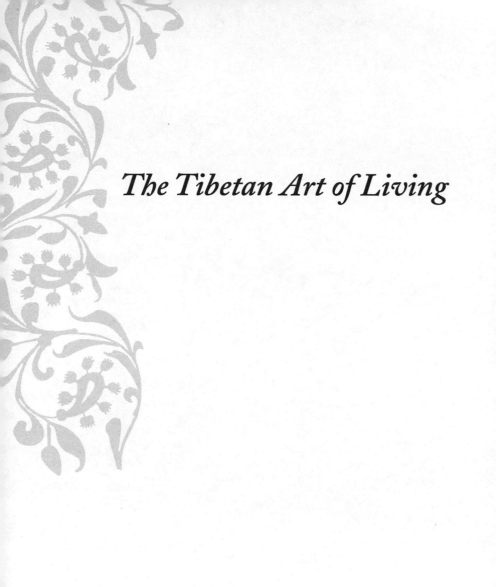

The Tibetan Art of Living

CHAPTER ONE

How Tibetan Wisdom Sees the World

This book is about how Tibetan medicine can help you to create wisdom, health, and well-being. It is not for scholars: There are already books of that kind by people well versed in the subject. This is primarily a book of self-exploration, which uses Tibetan medicine as a guide on the path to knowledge of your self.

We should regard ourselves as pilgrims following an inner journey that is beautiful, scary, and sometimes difficult. In these pages, you will learn about the art of living. You will discover many safe, traditional self-healing techniques that will empower you to become healthy and happy. Above all, you will experience the profound healing system within your being. Then, you can become your own best healer.

Understanding any culture can be difficult if you have not learned the thinking process behind it. It is the same with Tibetan medicine, which has its own special thinking process and language. In order for this book to be useful to you, it is important to know and experience the underlying worldview that is at the heart of one of the world's most sophisticated systems of healing.

Tibetan medicine is an ancient and detailed system that aims to unite the mind, body, and inner spirit of an ill person and so restore a dynamic balance. It works to create patterns of health by helping people change their mental and behavioral attitudes, even if the problem is a physical injury such as a broken leg. This does not mean that everything is in the mind. What Tibetan medicine does is to help people understand the origins and causes of illness, and how we hold illness in both our bodies and our minds.

By understanding why you are ill, why you have pain, why you suffer, you become stronger and wiser. You start to understand how and why any overwhelming or obstructive experience expresses itself as mental or physical illness. You then know how to stop suffering and heal both your illness and the way you live.

The Origins of Tibetan Dur Bön Medicine

Tibetan spirituality in all its forms goes back to a simple and basic belief held by the peoples of Tibet since the most ancient times. In order to gain spiritual growth you must first gain personal vitality and energy. This will make you strong and free from obstructions so that you attract only good things to you. This concept lies at the heart of all religious and spiritual thought of the Tibetan experience.

There are two structured religious teachings in Tibetan culture today. One is Buddhism and the other Bön, a Tibetan term that basically means "to invoke a deity." According to the Bön tradition, the great spiritual genius Tonpa Shenrab Miwo, who was born seventeen thousand years before the historical Buddha, founded the Bön teaching. As a fully enlightened person from birth, he was able to give teachings that helped people to cure their suffering.

Both Tonpa Shenrab Miwo and Buddha were regarded as master physicians because they diagnosed the root causes of suffering. They developed similar ideas about how to transform suffering, encourage happiness, and create inner balance. They understood the human condition.

The original practitioners of Dur Bön, from which my tradition developed, were married priests in pre-Buddhist times; their job was to prepare the bodies of dead kings and escort their souls to higher states of consciousness. They were advisers to royal families and important community leaders, and also held complex medical knowledge about how the body and mind worked and how it died and re-formed. This medical knowledge came from an older culture known as Zhang Zhung.

The Dur Bön school merged with a spiritual tradition known as dMu T'ang, which is also part of the Bön culture. In its earliest times dMu T'ang trained its exponents to send their minds into other realms of consciousness. This skill was used to heal, guide, and protect the community. The dMu T'ang tradition also held important spiritual and medical teachings in the forms of physical and mental exercises.

The practitioners of Dur Bön and dMu T'ang were mystics, philosophers, physicians, and scientists. Their legacy extended to all schools of Bön and has influenced Tibetan Buddhism as well. Rningmapa, the oldest school of Tibetan Buddhism, is similar to some aspects of Bön culture. Modern research suggests that many aspects of Indian and Chinese culture have borrowed much from Bön. The origins of Hinduism and the Taoist and feng shui philosophies of China all emanate from Bön culture and spirituality.

When Buddhism first came to Tibet in the seventh century A.D., it made little impact. In the eighth century, however, the government was in crisis and there was unrest among the Bön nobility. The Buddhists launched a well-planned military invasion and succeeded in becoming the dominant religion in Tibet until the Chinese invasion of 1959.

At first, the two systems of thinking—Buddhist and Bön—worked well together. Then, however, certain Buddhist factions started to persecute Bön communities. To stop the persecution, some Bön communities took on the trappings of the Buddhist teaching and developed into what became known as Reformed Bön, or *Bön-pos*. In reality, however, their teachings are much the same and there is little controversy between the two approaches. The search for virtue, compassion, and wisdom is the same for Buddhists as for all forms of Bön communities. My teacher, who was a Bön master and taught me the old Bön (the Bön of the Ngagpas), married a woman from a famous family of Buddhist teachers. He and his wife suffered no division in their spiritual practices or religious views.

His Holiness the Dalai Lama has recently taken a significant step in uniting the fabric of Tibet by acknowledging the crucial role of Bön in Tibetan culture. Those in the West who know anything about Bön tend to get it mixed up with indigenous Tibetan shamanism and animistic beliefs. This is inaccurate but, confusingly, both Buddhism and Bön endorse some, if not all, of those beliefs and have incorporated them into their way of thinking.

Indeed, all Tibetan teachings have succeeded in keeping their vitality and universal truths. Although Tibetan Buddhism is far better known today than Bön, there are still thousands of practitioners in Tibet and throughout the Himalayan region, and there are Bön religious communities in India, Eastern Tibet, North America, and some parts of Central Asia.

Currently, all religious activity in Tibet is outlawed. The

official religion today is the mindless adherence to Chinese Communism. But Buddhist and Bön communities are not the only ones to suffer from communist persecution. The Tibetan Muslims, Jews, and Christians have all suffered terribly.

How We See the World

According to Tibetan medicine, the body is a physical expression of mental energies generated by the brain. The nature of these energies is created by the way each person interprets the world around him.

Although we think that we are reacting instantaneously to everything that happens to us, we are, in fact, always living in the past, because our brains can only react through our senses. Consider this, and you'll see that your reaction is always a few seconds behind the event because of the time it takes to process via your senses and brain. Our sense of immediacy is an illusion. What we think is happening right now has already passed.

In the same way, illness creates an illusion about its nature, and it is this illusion that we need to see through. We are conditioned psychologically to expect to be ill. Because we live in this potent expectation, illness follows us like a stubborn dog that refuses to be sent home. Illness is a self-fulfilling prophecy.

HOW ILLNESS BUILDS UP IN OUR BODIES

Over time, extremely intense experiences, good or bad, slowly stun the body and mind. They infiltrate the central nervous system and leave their influence behind in the form of deeply rooted energies that abide in the deepest parts of the personality. Here, according to Tibetan medicine, these old influences build and create emotional and spiritual garbage that, in time, becomes physical and emotional illness or negative life circumstances.

These subtle underlying forces of ill health relate to "karma." The way we react to the stimuli around us and the illusion we have of living in the present create the causes and conditions of our lives. This is karma.

Karma can be defined as a conscious mental decision and action carried out for a particular end result. Every day we create karma by experiencing problems, coping with stress, eating or drinking too much, and even having too much of a good or bad time—when we are angry, lie, cause trouble for other people, or cause ourselves harm by acting before thinking things through. All of these daily experiences that we go through leave their imprints in our minds and bodies, on our lives and on those of other people. You will find a fuller explanation of karma in chapter 3.

How can we try to overcome this dilemma?

HEALTH IS A PROCESS

According to the Tibetans, health is like the tide. It is a process, not a static or constant experience. Each person's state of energy is continuously changing from one moment to the next, rising and falling, increasing and decreasing. When energy falls below a certain level, which differs from person to person, the first signs of illness are experienced.

Illness can take a long time to find its way into material form and may not be obvious. Many people go about their daily lives looking perfectly healthy on the outside, yet within they may have a deep-seated emotional problem or an unseen cancer carrying them closer to death. Some people allow stress, one of the most damaging influences on our health in modern times, to fester and build up inside so that years, even decades later, they find themselves burned out and ill.

To prevent the causes of illness you must know how to prevent unskillful patterns of emotions and behavior so that your life becomes more harmonious and balanced. You will meet the concept of skillful behavior frequently in this book. In a nutshell, skillful behavior leads to positive outcomes, unskillful to negativity.

Negativity and prejudice are closely related. People are united more by their prejudices—of every kind—than by any other common factor. Prejudice represses anyone who experiences it into a state of worthlessness and triviality. Illness can be seen as a prejudice that you have created toward yourself. By understanding how we think about ourselves, we learn how we create the foundations of health and illness and this in turn will show us how we create our own subconscious patterns of karma.

Your Life Is a Spiritual Experience

We see ourselves as flesh and blood, but, in fact, human beings are consciousness that has sought a way to express itself in this material world by taking on a physical form. Underneath all the physical and mental construction of daily life on this planet lies a pure and open spiritual consciousness. This is a natural state of mind that is always there within every person, entwined in the fabric of our lives.

This duality can create chaos and suffering. Illness is often brought about by our minds, emotions, and habits getting in the way of the pure consciousness at our core. But our innate spirituality can also create order and beauty.

Realizing that each of us has this infinite potential is at the heart of Tibetan spiritual teaching. It exists in everyone and everything. At this very moment, you are the great symbol of your own potential enlightenment.

The purpose of any spiritual practice, ethical framework, or religious belief should be to help us enjoy the lives that we have. What's important is to avoid getting caught up with the future, because the future—and the past—are only creations of our imaginations. To be happy we need first to allow ourselves to be so—now. So forget thoughts like "I will be so happy *if only* that would happen," and "I was so happy *when* things were different." All you have is now. So accept yourself as you are without embellishment or regret.

Start by aiming to experience everyday life in as open and direct a manner as possible. From the moment you wake to the moment you sleep, allow every experience to come to you without judgment. The key is acceptance.

Accepting whatever happens is a hard task at first. Like everyone, you will feel fear at the very idea, but gradually, as you cut through the barriers developed by years of habit, you will start to become less reactive to the world around you. We often live our whole lives in a state of reaction to experiences. If we are caused pain, we become angry, we hurt, we cry, we fear for our existence. These reactive responses continue the subtle links of our suffering. Whether they are big events in our lives or small ones, the end result is the same.

Acceptance takes the sting out of reactivity and creates for us insight into the way we make our lives happen. An experience of great simplicity will emerge from your consciousness as you allow acceptance to filter into all your mental and physical actions. It will make you feel naked and exposed at first, but, as you stay with this, you will learn that truth needs no clothing.

As you follow the path to your inner morality, many confused emotions may come to the surface of your everyday mind, causing you self-doubt and fear. You may worry that you are inferior to your colleagues and peers. Remember: You are not bad. You are essentially good, and intrinsically enlightened. You lack nothing. If you can accept this, the path will start to reveal itself.

Simply look at the natural world. Bees and flowers, clouds and rain, sun and moon, light and dark, birth and death—all of these are part of the continual cycle of truth. See how the ants and birds work together, each giving support to the others of their kind. Human beings often fail to do this. The seeds within the fruit know only one thing: that they must grow, blossom, and bear fruit. Essentially, we human beings must do the same, but some of us have forgotten. The truth is everywhere, in all things, in all situations, and is behind the beginning and completion of everything. It can lead you to your spiritual potential, and, most of all, it can reveal to you how to live your life.

Remember, living in a way that is as true to yourself as you can be is not always an easy path. Do not climb spiritual mountains just because they are there, or seek the meaning of life because you feel you should. *Life has only the meaning you give to it.* The truth reveals life as it is.

Spiritual Consciousness in the Twenty-first Century

The first one hundred years of the new millennium will dictate the cycles and patterns for the future. New forms of spiritual wisdom and consciousness are finding their roots. New technologies and the changes in the global economy and the use of natural resources will influence the evolution of human beings as a species.

Tibetan wisdom teaches that in this century, the foundations of the new wisdom will be manifested in the rising up of female and feminine consciousness, influencing both the worldview and individual development. This feminine consciousness will create new ways of thought, new insights into human nature, and will become humanity's next step on the evolutionary path to the understanding of its spiritual potential.

It can and will empower both men and women, redefining individual responsibility and revising our priorities. Individual and social spirituality will be the only important human resource that will guide us to the understanding of ourselves and our planet. People all over the world are starting to understand, deep within themselves, that the so-called modern world has not delivered. Although science and technology and rational philosophies have contributed to material and intellectual well-being, our spiritual needs are not being met.

Inner wisdom and higher states of consciousness form the only bedrock of individual spiritual happiness. They are the resonance of the higher humanity that links all people. But we feel separated from them. In this troubled time, careful understanding of the past, present, and future can bring great insight.

Many people understand that life on our planet is simply a transition to a higher level. But often we have closed down those very perceptions that can reveal to us our inner light, and so we stay confined to this world and its material emanations. The risk is that if we do not reach out now for whatever we see as heaven or higher consciousness, then hell and hellish states of mind will slowly creep upon us.

The earth is going through a painful adolescence, for not only is humanity a young species but so is the rock on which we live. We are living in a kind of global puberty. Squeezed between the old and the new, we forget the constant that is there regardless of history, time, or politics: our ability both as individuals and as a species to reconnect with one another and with the gifts of nature. For this we need to allow our humility to emerge. Humility is the foundation of generosity.

To find this humility, you must encourage simplicity of thought and directness of action in all parts of your life. Respect the society that you find yourself in and understand that great value can be found in what you have and are. Most people can understand and experience their spiritual potential without any particular training. A focused and sincere heart and a direct mental focus are often enough. The purpose is simply to comprehend the underlying spiritual nature of all things. From this develops a way of manifesting freedom, peace, happiness, and higher consciousness.

All of us are wise. All of us have access to inner truth. No one holds a single key to truth above all others. Rest in your emerging divinity and consciousness. Do not grasp for it. Receive it and enjoy.

Live every day not as if it were your last, but for what it is: an unknown experience, potentially able to offer you a connection to your humanity and happiness. We need to realize that the process of traveling toward our dreams is in itself a spiritual experience.

In the next chapter you will discover how to create your soul for this life, a process the Tibetan Bön tradition calls Activating Your Thunder, because the individual who has made his or her soul has the power of thunder and lightning to cut through ignorance and reveal truth to others.

CHAPTER TWO

Activating Your Thunder—How to Make Your Soul and Keep It

The soul is not eternal. A soul lasts for a lifetime and through the process of dying. Then it breaks down—a spiritually biodegradable process of the mind. So we are not reborn complete with a soul, but we do come to this life with all the ingredients to make one.

Each of us is a being with many dimensions, all working together simultaneously. As we start to explore these inner dimensions, in the process of building our souls for this life, we begin to know a little of the vastness and complexity of our consciousness. The soul is a device that holds and directs our consciousness and potential enlightenment. Regardless of our backgrounds, each of us is a beginner when it comes to building one. It's important to remember that there is no test to be passed, no degree to be gained, no point of perfection to be attained. The process is an experience that comes from understanding the energy within ourselves and all other living things.

Let me clear up one common area of confusion: We are never completely what we imagine ourselves to be—either good or bad. This is because our view of ourselves and our lives is made up primarily of the reactive emotions that I mentioned in chapter 1. These egocentric feelings, generated in the battle of everyday living, often loop around like a psychic tape, replaying the same experiences within us. We may become addicted to a particular emotion that makes us feel good in some way. Don't get me wrong: Emotions are important and valuable, but we should not let them fool us into believing that they are life or consciousness.

Most of what we consider to be our identity is the shadows of past habits and sensory overload. By starting to understand the nature of our habits, which form the everyday mind, we begin to be able to unite all these separate inner forces on the first step to creating our souls. It is then that we gain a vision of who we really are.

Love is essential to our humanity and thus to our souls. Love is experienced as a means of understanding the nature of existence and the transient nature of possessions—people or objects—and suffering, as well as the unalterable process of karma.

Tibetan thought reminds us to show real care, love, and compassion in all that we do and think to the best of our ability and intellect. Love for ourselves and others—in any context, experience, or form—passionately involves itself in every living being, holding all things within its own calm cradle of respect and nonjudgment. True love always wants the best for every creature in existence, loving all the world without prejudice but with wisdom.

Nonattachment is an aspect of loving wisely and involves being joyful in the joy of others. In simple terms, it means no-strings-attached love, without expectation or obligation. Love is often interwoven with some form of attachment, but in Tibetan thought, this is firmly discouraged. Attachment has connotations of expectation, need, and even greed. When you love without attachment, you do so selflessly, without any expectation of reward. You simply love.

In Tibetan teachings you do not reject the world, you embrace it. You become intimate with life. The single acceptable and healthy type of attachment is attachment to your inner devotion and development. Attachment to the divine in yourself can inspire a real human love for everyone, which is truly remarkable. Consider how many people you love and are attached to: friends, partners, and even to enemies; teachers, relatives, neighbors, and co-workers; celebrities of all kinds, and not least to your pets. The list goes on and on. Ask yourself, "What is the nature of my attachment?" Many of these relationships can be positive tools for transformation, although they may also carry some threads of expectation and obligation that you might want to unravel.

We need also to look at the attachments we have to our physical bodies. We may have a love affair with them or feel trapped in them, hate them or be anxious about them. We must learn to let go of any negative feelings with kindness so that we can relate to our bodies in a new and loving way. Similarly, we must learn to look beyond the concept that our bodies are our identities.

Whenever our capacity for love is great, so is our capacity for suffering. Through suffering we learn the timeless value of love. When we lose someone we care for through separation or death, we grieve and suffer, but from that attachment comes knowledge. If we value the experience of true grief, we can learn and move on. It is better to accept suffering in its totality than to embrace the prejudice-creating concept of inhuman composure.

Spirituality of any type should bring you closer to your humanity. If you end up cold and cut off, without emotional understanding, you have, through your perception of holiness, committed an act of spiritual terrorism both to yourself and other people. The further we remove ourselves from others the more we are lost. The more detached we become from our humanity, the more powerful our egos become. Be human first, middle, and last. That is where divinity is to be found.

This process of soul-making is creation of the highest type because we become the creators of our connection to a greater reality. It is vital that we learn to build strong souls that can withstand the storms of everyday living.

In this chapter we will learn about the nature of consciousness, the physical and mental vitality we need to start building a soul, the five spiritual foundations of the soul, and how to develop our five senses.

This is the story of how I started to create my soul.

It was a summer evening on Mount Pihanga in the center of the North Island of New Zealand.

The evening sky stood bright and strong against the night. Everything was still; there was no wind, no breeze. The lake below was placid, reflective. The mountain above stood strong, defiant, and knowing.

"Tonight we shall start learning to make a soul," said Ürgyen, my teacher. "We are all born without a soul, but most people do not know how to create one. You must first look at the energy of the soul. Observe."

He gazed out across the valley. Everything became even more still than before. He raised his right hand into the air, his palm facing out into the night. He started to chant, slow and long, and everything in front of me burst into light and clear flame. My jaw hit my knees; a part of me could not believe what I saw. But my doubt faded as I looked closer: the sky, the stars, the trees, the air, mountain, lake, and the hill I was on had become an incandescent flame. Then I looked down at myself: I too was part of this flame.

"This is the energy from which all things are made," said

Ürgyen. "It is consciousness. It is you and I, and all living creatures. It is this energy that forms our minds and our souls."

Suddenly it was gone. The stars, the mountain, and the lake were as they had been before.

My teacher explained that our senses are devices that interpret what is going on *around* us in the everyday world. Less obviously, they also interpret what is going on *within* us in the everyday world. Crucially, it is this spiritual dimension to our senses that allows our minds to connect with the energy that pulses in the hearts of other living creatures and in the essence of inanimate existence, from grains of sand on the seashore to vast oceans. You will learn the importance of interconnectedness in this chapter and at the end there are exercises to help you develop your senses.

Every living thing is connected. Human beings, for instance, live in one another's consciousness more intimately than most people care to acknowledge. The main factors that influence and transform our senses, and which we can use in building a soul, are set out in this ancient Tibetan Bön saying:

Thought is the body of Sound.
Sound is the body of Light.
Light is the body of Consciousness.
Consciousness is the body of humanity.
The soul, once made, is the body of these.

Thought and Sound

Our thoughts are our individual distillations of the sounds of the world and the universe—of mankind, of nature, of life living itself. These sounds fill the broad spectrum of life and find their expression in human thought, which then leads to creativity and endeavor.

Sound and Light

According to ancient Tibetan belief, sound is made up of light. Light, both physical and spiritual, is the essence of the construction of all sound.

The entwining of sound and light are apparent in music, perhaps the most powerful and universal form of art. Inner light can drive forward sounds that form part of our personal environment, and the opposite is also true. From a Tibetan view, the music to which we are attracted actually creates light within our brains and nervous systems and encourages spiritual light to shine within our consciousness.

Music, as well as other forms of art, is often an expression of the mental forces of humanity at any given time, as well as a reflection of the psychic health of our planet. This is because the works are full of light and sound—in other words, consciousness. Think of composers such as Mozart, Beethoven, and Bach, and painters like Picasso and Matisse.

However dramatic they may seem at the time, shifts and changes in our world, as a result of wars, natural disasters, disease, and even pornography and pop music, are a natural part of the cycles of our planet as it floats in the universe.

Light and Consciousness

The essence of light is consciousness, whether it's physical energy—from the sun, the moon, a fire, even a light bulb—or inner spiritual energy. This consciousness is the summation of all physical and spiritual energies coming together. When you have made your soul, you will gain insight into the interrelationships between what people separate as spiritual or physical. You will understand that, in fact, they are the same energy expressed in different forms. When you truly accept this, you will find that the world gladly reveals itself in all its dimensions of existence.

Consciousness

Consciousness is our essence. It is the energy that creates everything in the universe.

Consciousness expresses itself in different ways. Our evolution as a physical species is wrapped around this consciousness. Think of the words *spiritual, spirit, and inspiration,* and compare them to the process that keeps our physical bodies alive—respiration. At its most fundamental, every breath we take is a physical expression of consciousness. Later in the book you will find some breathing exercises.

Consciousness does not change, nor does it stand still. It is the root of evolution. Very old Bön texts talk of a time millions of years ago when the world was young and covered in great cycles of floods. People lived in caves or on high mountains, yet they had the same consciousness as we do today. But the underlying consciousness, which exists in all things, is always slowly finding ways of evolving into broader and more profound dimensions. Without this process, we would not, for instance, be able to study our emotions, intellect, and spirituality. The evolution of consciousness is what enables us to make a soul.

It is by creating the soul that you go from becoming reactive and controlled by both your emotional and physical environments into a state of consciousness in which you become the originator of your life, understanding the flux and flow of consciousness and knowing how to use it.

Now let us look at the cultural background in Tibetan teaching that helped develop the spiritual and psychological techniques of making a soul.

Origins

As mentioned previously, Tibetan culture and spirituality originated in the shamanism of Central and Northern Asia. These cultures taught sophisticated theories of the mind, spiritual meditations, and other techniques that connected the individual to a transcendent joy and a natural happiness.

A happy spiritual life was seen as a balance of spiritual and material activities. The first step was that you, as an individual, had to become empowered by making and keeping your soul. This meant that your life force, mental clarity, and overall inner state needed to be stronger than the world around you. This included the worlds of thoughts and emotions as well as the material world and the environment.

THEN AND NOW

Tibetan shamans (Ngagpas), like those from other cultures, sought to create a balance between humankind and the forces of nature. Nature in all its manifestations was deeply respected as the organ of the health of our planet by Ngagpas. With today's environmental crisis and the new illnesses and diseases affecting the global community, it is crucial for all human beings to rediscover the relationships and harmonies central to shamanistic wisdom. In this way, the earth can be healed, repaired, and managed, and humankind can be saved from worldwide negativity, social decline, and individual suffering. If we keep polluting our planet, we end up polluting ourselves, emotionally, physically, and, eventually, spiritually.

If we develop a direct knowledge of our human consciousness and use it skillfully as we interact with all dimensions of life, we can achieve power and balance in our own lives and harmony for the earth.

Building Blocks of the Gods

Ngagpas experience the divine essence in humanity on a daily basis. This can be true for each of us, but we are not consciously aware of it. We are all made from the building blocks of god-energies and it is in our power to find the optimum situations for happiness and spiritual awakening.

The Ngagpas' role is to restore the natural harmonies that existed at the very first heartbeat of all humanity. Ngagpas create wise connections between all forms of consciousness, the forces of the natural world, those of the cosmos and other realms, and those of the earth in all its forms and variations.

This role is something that all human beings instinctually know and respond to. If we deny it, we deny ourselves. We are all Ngagpas in some way, within the personal context of our own lives. These skills come from discipline of the mind and body but they also derive from, and are grown by, the conscious creation and construction of a soul.

SOUL ENERGY AND THE CREATION OF VITALITY

According to Tibetan wisdom, making a soul is dependent on having vitality. This is the life force that feeds us and gives us drive. The storehouse of vitality is created during our conception and activated during the physical birth event. It is crucial to the health of our bodies and minds—indeed, to our very existence as emotional, energetic, and spiritual beings.

But this vital energy can become depleted by the ups and downs of life and may be unable to renew itself. When this happens, illness, suffering, unhappiness, bad fortune, or severe obstructions come into our lives and the concept of creating a soul seems irrelevant.

21

Depleted vitality tries to renew itself, but the process may become distorted and result in the creation of further obstructions and problems that come back again and again, just as you think you have finally dealt with them.

It may be difficult to restore strong vitality, but it can be done. Knowing more about your personal history is the first step in restoring dwindling vitality. Think about the low points in your life and study, for example, what time of year they happened, what kinds of people were around you at the time, and what those people meant to you. You will discover that there are cycles in your life, highs and lows, that correspond to the rise and fall of your vitality. Often, because our vitality is unstable and fragile, we have very fast rises and falls, which are preludes to a series of repetitive problems, situations, and obstructions. Examining these cycles will help you to understand the nature of your depleted vitality and how it happened.

The aim is not to create more vitality—you are born with a finite amount—but to improve the quality of your vital force, making it stronger and more durable. Treating yourself with respect and balance improves and restores vitality, facilitates the flow of happiness and good fortune, and enables you to set about the process of making a soul.

Vitality and the Art of Living Well

It's important to remember that living well is not only a skill but an art, which involves three main factors: other people, yourself, and vitality. If you wish to practice the art, you must understand its components. Ancient Tibetan tradition teaches that there are nine types of activities, all of which are intimately connected with our physical, emotional, and psychological states of vitality.

The nine types of vital activity concern:

1. Food and diet

2. Behavior

3. Work/career

4. Inner world

5. Spiritual needs and beliefs

6. Generosity and compassion

7. Mental discipline

8. Happiness

9. Sharing, giving, and receiving

In the chapters that follow, you will find detailed information about these vital activities and how you can best nourish them. For now, here is a brief introduction to what they are and how they affect your life.

1. Food and Diet

Food is energy and it gives greater or lesser types of vitality to your system, depending on how you use it. Tibetan medicine is concerned not just with eating "healthy" foods but with eating the right types of food for your physical and psychological type. If you eat foods that are not compatible with your type, your vitality becomes dispersed and weak.

Now let us take a brief look at dieting. The Western world has gone diet mad. Dieting can be good for you, but if done incorrectly it damages your health and weakens your psychological and physical vitality in a very powerful way. When you start to diet, you change the way your body and mind work through the subtle restrictions you exercise on your attitudes and ideas, including the merits of different foods, your physical reaction to those foods, and your body image.

Restricting what you eat is of real benefit only when you are ill. If you diet just to lose weight, the weight will return in some form. For dieting to be beneficial in the long term, there must be life-style changes that empower both your body and your mind. A sensible diet is a good way of fine-tuning the overall health of your body. It should be undertaken for one month once every two years, in early to mid-January, to improve your vitality.

Alcohol is an ancient and socially accepted drug, so its abuse is very easy. It is good to reduce your alcohol intake to a level where it brings you occasional pleasure rather than constant remorse. If you drink a lot, you deplete your vitality. Coffee can act in a similar way if it is abused. Like alcohol, caffeine is a complex drug whose abuse has created global social problems, particularly with the proliferation of caffeinated drinks. Drinking more water is wise for everyone but is particularly important to counterbalance the effects of these drinks. The Tibetan approach to food and drink is outlined fully in chapter 8.

2. Behavior

This concerns the way you react to others and to circumstances. All human beings, regardless of how they may seem, are intrinsically fragile. The older we become, the more fragile we get.

One of the most important aspects of behavior is speech and the thoughts behind it. Negative thoughts and speech diminish vitality and so diminish us. If you react in an unloving way to people, you transfer your difficulties to them. Behaving in this way can easily become a habit and cause suffering both to you and to the people with whom you communicate. By learning how your mind works and reacts on a day-to-day basis (what I call your "everyday mind"), you will learn not to harm your fragile emotional and physical state or that of anyone else.

If you get a bad reaction from someone, you invariably pass it on. This is where the majority of people cause themselves and others the most pain, which decreases their vitality. This happens because deep within every human being is an honest and heartfelt desire to communicate and to interact with others in a friendly and kind way. When we are treated "badly," as we see it, we feel let down and abused. Thus, our aim is to be unaffected by rejection, rudeness, or unkindness, and to help others to achieve the same immunity.

Vitality has a personality of its own, which seeks to expand and blend with everything, from rocks and stars to people and animals. Though it may not be obvious to us, it is this impulse that causes us to seek communication with one another, to be creative, and to aspire to the highest dimensions of human intelligence. Misused, however, this impulse can be gruesome and evil, causing us to seek dominion over others.

3. Work/Career

Work is any activity that involves people communicating with one another, so it is a vast part of human life. In these situations, there is always an exchange of vitality among people, and it is a natural process. According to Tibetan wisdom, the essential reason for all human work is to interact with others and to experience a heightened vitality. This experience in turn creates the work and its end result.

Often in the workplace or in your career, however, you will experience fatigue and a loss of vitality. This comes not from the activity but how you react to it, and also from the way you communicate with others and they with you. Tibetan teaching has always suggested that in any form of human activity or endeavor you achieve your aims with other people helping you. But you need to be watchful because while some people can increase or stabilize your vitality, others can reduce it.

You need to recognize when your vitality is being abused, either consciously or unconsciously. Conversely, if you feel empowered by other people, you need to work out how you can best handle it. Vital force is an intimate aspect of our individuality within the everyday world and it is our personal responsibility to look after it.

Our attitude to work is key. Many people think of it only as a means to pay for our lives—that work is something we have to do in order to make money or be part of society. This is partly true, of course, but if you work with this attitude in mind, your vitality will certainly diminish. Also, the workplaces we choose and/or the career goals we set for ourselves are often highly effective devices for reducing the potency of our vitality, or even cutting us off from our connection to it.

Constructive attitudes toward work can build up your vitality. Anything you do can be perceived as a way for your consciousness to learn and grow. Work shows us our limitations but also our qualities and talents. It can make us more emotionally mature, which allows us to become less affected by negative work environments or unskillful people.

Yes, many places of work are negative. For instance, you may be physically injured or be victimized by office politics, or simply be stuck in a mediocre organization. Remember that the workplace is often where we discover the nature of karmic forces, for human nature is shown there in all its guises. By overcoming such problems we are able to connect with our inner vitality. Remember, too, that workplaces and your career have their own special vital force, which you will begin to recognize as you make contact with your vitality.

Last, if you find you cannot practice your spiritual beliefs in your workplace, you must revisit what you believe, because that area of your vitality is weak.

4. Inner World

Your inner world is a place of secrets, dreams, hopes, aspirations, fantasies, and plans—of longing, anger, love, hope, ambition, and the yearning for happiness. This inner place can be both a sanctuary and a place of turmoil. It is where vitality withers or flourishes because here we create our deepest identity through our desires. Your vitality takes on the qualities of the dominant emotional forces that are active deep within you. These are the true forces that feed your everyday persona.

Vitality is intrinsically pure, all-encompassing, and life-giving. But we can pollute it by repeated unskillful actions and thoughts, such as abusing our bodies through drugs or other behaviors that cause us and other people hurt, pain, or confusion. So each of us needs to be aware of the nature of our inner world. Is it really the place you want to be? Are you happy there?

Our inner world sets up the way in which we relate to the world around us. It guides us to all of the achievements and successes in our lives. It is the inner world that decides our needs and desires as they really are, because our inner world is who we really are.

Without an inner world that functions in an integrated way, you do not have a life, simply an experience of living spattered by periods of unknowing, powerlessness, and the sudden need for control. When life seems more powerful than you do, your inner world needs healing.

Nearly all of us pass our lives floating on top of our inner world, sublimely unconscious of just how unknowing and how lacking in personal empowerment we really are. Yet, if we have the courage to explore within, we will discover among the fear and anger an endless beauty, an eternal light that shines from within us out into a world and universe of endless possibilities. At the core of our inner world beats an endless love that needs no language or intelligence to be understood, just a heart that is ready to be humble.

5. Spiritual Needs and Beliefs

A spiritual belief is quite different from a spiritual need. A spiritual belief enables you to understand a truth in your own way. A spiritual need enables you to live, to be alive. Needs are basic and instinctual, the staple diet of the consciousness that makes us human. All of us have spiritual needs that are determined by the way that we have lived since conception. If, as individuals, we do not find a way to fulfill these needs, our lives are incomplete and we become ill.

Spiritual needs fall into three basic groups:

1. The need for a reality of belonging, safety, and harmony

2. The need for a reality of happiness, beauty, and achievement

3. The need for a reality of continuity, wisdom, and unconditional love

In this new millennium, people have needs, not beliefs. Because this new century is the template for those to come, people are and will continue to be under increasing psychic pressure. The way in which this pressure can be released is through the fulfillment of spiritual needs. The vitality that comes from this is the anchor of all of the nine activities.

The vitality of spiritual need unites all living creatures in a common inheritance of life and living. By cultivating it through self-knowledge, you become more human; that is, you become connected to the divinity that exists in the daily experience of living. By knowing the beauty that upholds the functions of everyday life, you will discover that ordinary events and situations hold the key to experiencing your spiritual beauty and perfection.

In the search for self-knowledge, the greatest adventure that any person can undertake is the voyage within. You do not need to look outside your life to find greater truths, because every day of your life is an enormous state of grace that holds lessons about your true nature. Spiritual development is just like the act of living and dying; no one can prepare you for the process, you learn as you go along. All you need is the courage to start.

The one thing that everyone needs on his or her spiritual journey is the quality of acceptance. This is the greatest survival tool of all, a spiritual Swiss army knife, because it teaches you adaptability, patience, and good humor. These three qualities make your life enjoyable, give perspective to all your experiences, and help you to assess and treasure your vitality.

6. Generosity and Compassion

Generosity and compassion are the two structures of life that hold it together. They are the underpinning of all good things. Without them our lives have no vitality; they are merely shadows, sick, empty, and one-dimensional.

Generosity is not just the act or mental attitude of giving, it is also a way of living that creates abundance for everyone else. Generosity is life-giving.

Compassion, however, is life-making. It is a transformational state of consciousness that gives new life to all beings who consider themselves defeated by the events of their lives.

Compassion is the foundation and identity of humanity. By showing compassion as best we can, we become more evolved and more integrated. This creates an enduring wisdom, the nature of which is generosity of spirit. This in turn becomes happiness.

7. Mental Discipline

Mental discipline is the first step toward lasting happiness. You need mental discipline to understand and appreciate your happiness. When people are happy but do not understand why, they often misuse their happiness. Then vitality is diminished and happiness cannot be supported, so it vanishes.

If we know why and how we are happy, we can create more happiness for ourselves, and that means more vitality. This is the start of mental discipline. Mental discipline is not a strict, regimented control of the way in which your mind deals with facts by routine or planned structure; it is a state of wisdom.

This wisdom comes not from knowledge or intellect—factual information is memory, not wisdom—but from an openness that expands your emotional and spiritual awareness. Ignorance is generated when your mind is closed or will not accept new influences in your life.

The wiser people become, the freer they are from anger, delusion, hatred, possessiveness, and all forms of prejudice. They become totally receptive to all offerings from life. They are receptive but also discerning.

There is a danger of creating a false mental discipline through adherence to religion rather than spirituality. It is here that we should explore a little more the nature of the senses. We must learn to value our senses and the experiences they bring to us. We must respect them so that their gifts can grow in intensity and depth. From this they become clear and shine with the light that streams out of total realization.

Our senses allow our inner essence to unfold and from this comes originality, beauty, and the sparks of perception. Sight, sound, smell, touch, taste, and all other physical sensations connect us all to one another's experience of humanity. This connection is the way to unity, to understanding that each human being on the planet today is a link to the experience of enlightenment. As we discover this, a spiritual echo starts to vibrate on a frequency within our inner minds that excites us to search for meaning.

If we do not go through this process for ourselves but only pick up the echo, we construct a religion rather than a spiritual experience. Religion alone is a false mental discipline that can become rigid and unbending. Both in history and the world today there are many examples of religious intolerance, violence, and corruption created out of false mental discipline.

True mental discipline is free of ego. It is not a denial of who you are, but an understanding of how your mind works, how it supports you—and how it tricks you. The more you can discipline and direct your mental forces, the better the quality of mental experience you will have. It will create wisdom and generate awareness and a happiness that survives within you regardless of what happens in your daily life.

8. Happiness

We have discussed happiness a lot in previous sections because it is so important. Most people equate happiness with an obvious absence of suffering. This is not happiness, but a lack of problems. Often, however, we do not believe that there is a deeper happiness.

A deeper happiness does exist, if we take the trouble to cultivate it. We can grow happiness inside us. Just like crops, true happiness must be planted from seed, grown, harvested, and made into a useful creation. Cultivating this particular vitality is one of the purposes of having a human existence. People who have the vitality of happiness bring happiness to all living creatures just by the very fact that they exist. Happiness is the greatest form of beauty that we can experience.

Happiness also keeps us healthy. If a patient consults a physician of Tibetan medicine about a lack of vitality, the first thing he or she will do is to discover if the person is happy or not, and why. When just one person is unhappy, all of humankind is affected in lesser or greater ways. With today's global media, we know that millions of people are very unhappy every day, and this affects all of us.

Our perception of happiness and suffering is sometimes ill-founded. If you have ever dealt with people who experience ongoing suffering, year in and year out, you know that under their fatigue lives a beauty and a happiness. You know that suffering does not go on forever. You know, too, that however they are feeling, happiness can come at any time and embrace them, rekindling their humanity. I have seen it happen in war zones and in the sickbeds of the First World. It is something we should not forget.

The erratic vitality of our human species has caused a deep lack of communal vitality across the world, which has resulted in war, famine, disease, and climate change. If we were able to restore the vital force of loving kindness to the world, the collective burden that we unconsciously share would start to lift. Our mental and emotional faculties would be transformed. It would take some considerable time, but all of us can start to contribute a little by knowing ourselves. As our vitality grows, the terrible situations that millions of people experience will start to improve.

Suffering takes on many forms and has much to teach us. When we consider other people's experiences, we know that happiness is never far from us. It is everywhere, in all things. It bubbles under the surface of our daily lives, waiting for us to recognize it in ourselves.

9. Sharing, Giving, and Receiving

These three activities can determine the outcome of our own personal humanity. Yet we tend to forget them as a form of communication because they take place at every minute of our daily lives. How much we give, receive, and share determines our abilities to understand ourselves.

The vitality generated by giving without expectations helps to heal the mind of agitation and encourages physical health both in the giver and the receiver. Sharing skillfully acknowledges that we are all caretakers of what we have or own, and that resources—great or small—are to be enjoyed but also respected, ready to pass on to new caretakers. Receiving is the hardest aspect of this vitality. To receive well requires a state of humility where we can accept the individual who gives something to our consciousness. We also need to be able to distinguish when this is beneficial to us and when it is not.

The art of skillful receiving generates currents of positive energy that flow throughout the world, creating generosity, material abundance, and cultural and scientific progress. We are all involved in the generation of these good things, so each one of us is responsible for all aspects of the planet, as a caretaker and guide to its evolution.

As well as being caretakers for the planet, we are caretakers and guides for ourselves. This means that we need to treat ourselves with more generosity through giving, sharing, and, most important, receiving human kindness. There is no greater experience in any person's life than to be treated with genuine human kindness. It is an act of grace that transforms us all and that all of us are able to share in. Beneath the masks of everyday living, this state of grace is who we really are.

The Five Foundations of the Soul

Just as your house needs foundations, so does your soul. The bricks and mortar of the soul are five forms of intelligence that you can integrate into your daily life to form your spiritual energy and power.

1. Experience the knowing behind your senses.

2. Experience inner silence.

3. Learn to listen.

4. Understand the nature of free will and the interconnection among all things.

5. Accept that consciousness is in everyone and everything.

The benefits of building these foundations are immense. They are traditionally regarded as the five aspects of consciousness that become developed as we create our soul potential. You will find these benefits explained in the following pages along with descriptions of the foundations. I have described my experiences of learning some of the foundations because it is the simplest way to explain.

A Request

The world made by human beings often demands a great deal from each of us. These demands can cause us to treat our lives without much respect. This is the nature of unconnected living. The universe, the natural world, and our inner con-

sciousness make no such demands. The inner world, the natural world, and the universe make only one request and there is plenty of time to hear it.

The request is this: You are already in a state of grace and balance. You are already awake to the potential of your consciousness. Please accept this as so and it shall take place.

Listen. All of this is closer than you think. Enlightenment is already blazing within you. It does not matter who you are or what you have done. Be humble enough to love yourself and then you can move forward.

THE FIRST FOUNDATION: EXPERIENCE THE KNOWING BEHIND YOUR SENSES

My breathing was heavy and my lungs felt as if they were being beaten by a sledgehammer. My heart banged loudly in my head. Thunder from the nearby mountain yelled defiance across the valley, lightning streaked across the peaks. Then everything stopped.

Silence.

Then the absence of silence.

A blue flickering light ran through me. It burned to white. The white turned to the sound of the ocean. A gentle humming started in my physical heart, then started to move in a spiral throughout my body. Each note was a little pearl of sound. Each pearl was connected to the next on a thread. The thread was me, formed of my burned desires and fearfulness, of wonder and discipline, of divinity and consciousness.

The making of my soul had begun.

The spiral stretched through all my bones, moving into the sacred part of my brain where, according to Tibetan beliefs, the potential for soul-making sleeps. The world around me was me. As the wind blew, so did I. As a stranger died, so did I.

And I knew that there were no strangers in our lives, only distant relatives to whom we have not yet been introduced.

I could feel the structures of my mind link with my body. My nervous system was my thinking process, which became a fuse of burning consciousness, like a flaming beacon in a desert. Within me I saw the inner tree, the burning bush described by the Ngagpas.

The tree was the vital channels of the mental body joining with the physical to create the soul. My senses started to transform. Each one became a form of intelligence, all five working together to hold my consciousness, to form my spiritual energy and power.

Benefits: Material

As you develop this energy, you will find that problems concerning money, relationships, career, and health start to improve. You will begin to learn about the nature of material energy and the most auspicious times in which to create financial and material success. You will begin to understand the essential nature of the relationships around you. You will either want to start a new, more fulfilling career or reappraise your current occupation. You will begin to recognize how all of these activities affect your physical and mental health and this will help you to improve your vitality.

THE SECOND FOUNDATION: EXPERIENCE INNER SILENCE

Ürgyen gazed at the fire, drinking tea. Everything was filled with the roar of divinity. But there was silence. No wind. No crackling from the fire, no loud thoughts, no thunder on the mountain.

I knew I was looking into the world of the everyday mind

through the eyes of my new soul. Then, with a roar of nature, it all returned: the wind blew, the fire crackled, thunder crashed around the mountain.

Ürgyen looked up. "The second foundation of building a soul is to be in the silence."

From the mountain across the valley came a peal of thunder and a flash of sheet lightning. The full moon hung over the mountain peak, watching.

Silence is a process, not a sound. It is something we must work to understand. Silence is an important faculty of human consciousness. Silence allows the consciousness to expand, and all the rubbish of our minds and personalities to fall away, so we can see ourselves a little more clearly. It reveals to us whether we like our own company or not.

The more time we spend in the company of silence, the more we are able to understand the mental and physical structures for inner change. To grow we need to be unafraid of silence. If we regard it only as the absence of noise, it can be overwhelming. Silence is the still point within all sound and motion. Just as a tornado has a still center, so silence is at the center of all things. The more we understand silence, the more we know about listening, about speech, and about thought. Silence is seen as the first step to thinking well.

Like most things in our lives, silence must be experienced to be understood. Most of us have very little silence in our lives, because our minds are too busy banging away at everyday affairs to stop and experience silence. You cannot be silent but silence can be within you.

If you discover the silence within, your life will change. You will want something else, something more fulfilling. Possibly your current life-style will taste stale, outmoded. Alternatively, it could suddenly become more enriched and improve beyond recognition.

Fulfillment is not truth or happiness. Fulfillment in this

context means a completion of activities and emotions, the natural end to a process of understanding. Fulfillment can come to you by allowing the silence within to manifest itself.

Benefits: Mental and Emotional

Your mental abilities will become more structured and comprehensive; you will be able to marry intuition with your everyday life to have a truly creative mental dimension. Problem-solving will become easier. Access to your intellectual skills will be easier and you will also understand the origins of your emotions. Understanding how our emotions work and how they form the instinctual part of us inspires us to treat our emotional personalities with more respect.

THE THIRD FOUNDATION: LEARN TO LISTEN

Hearing and listening are very different activities. Hearing is instinctual, a process of active consciousness that enables us to comprehend the world around us and to understand what we hear. Hearing comes from the everyday mind.

Listening is a spiritual skill whereby you can become the same as whatever you are listening to, and know its essence. Listening activates the essential qualities of what is being listened to, whether that is a person or anything else. Listening goes beyond using your ears; all your other senses connect and become involved, too.

Listening with an open heart creates relaxation, good health, and recognition of consciousness on both sides. Most of all, true listening is a mark of respect and compassion for whatever you listen to.

Listening is the key to the body's lock. Consciousness is the door that opens if you have learned how to listen well. Listen to the wisdom and energy of your body and you will know that, like the mind, the body moves in cycles that can guide you to transformation.

Benefits: Intellectual

Your intellectual abilities will start to improve and you will be able to grasp intellectual aspects of your own mind and apply them. The development of intellectual skills is an important aspect of a balanced spiritual wisdom.

Intellect can be used to help you understand and achieve happiness. You can achieve happiness by using reason, logic, examination, and discernment to observe the nature of how people suffer.

As you do this, you start to equate what you have seen with your experiences of suffering and those of other people. Because you are a human being, you are able to work out the cause of your suffering. This is a great ability, but one that many people do not use.

It is through your intellect that spiritual and emotional growth must express themselves, so you will then have an intellectual understanding of an inner experience that is, for the most part, beyond words. Mental discipline is important here because it helps you to value what you have made.

THE FOURTH FOUNDATION: UNDERSTAND THE NATURE OF FREE WILL AND THE INTERCONNECTION AMONG ALL THINGS

Because we are physically alive, emotionally active, and spiritually aware, this foundation is an ongoing experience that is with us all our lives in differing forms of development.

It can be developed through many different means. Free will starts as a product of ignorance but can become a tool of the wise. Free will is at work when we act in ignorance and do something—big or small, thought or deed—without knowing the consequences.

As we grow in consciousness, however, and know more about the possible interactions of thoughts, actions, and events, our will becomes free in a different way, because it becomes more informed. At this juncture, we know our responsibilities to all other living creatures. Then it is up to us to decide to live as we choose.

There is an interconnection among all things. By simply trying to listen to it, appreciate it, and understand it as much as you are able, you will attract its energy. That will support you and bring you to an experience that leads to the benefits explained below. Happiness comes from knowing of and experiencing your interconnection with all people on this planet. It comes from taking responsibility for creating your own happiness, then sharing that with others.

Benefits: Emotional

You will experience the dynamic nature of emotions and how they nurture and feed everything that makes us human, as both physical and spiritual beings. The origins of all our emotional patterns, habits, desires, preferences, and prejudices can be discovered and understood.

Emotional energy is the force that connects us to the cycles of nature and to other instinctual forces within humanity. By making a soul, you move beyond the limitations of instinct into the experience of empathy. Empathy is educated and disciplined intuitive energy of such refinement and loving power that you can identify with other people. They experience your doing so, which brings them hope and healing. Many people can do this in different ways. Perhaps you can. Try. In such things we are all novices because it is an experience that we must constantly relearn and reexperience.

Instinct is not bad, but it can be indulgent, because it is conditioned by the everyday mind. Empathy is the desire to connect with other people with unreserved compassion tempered by discernment. As people become empathetic because of their own life experiences and the inner exploration of their consciousness, they become less dominated by the negativities of instinct. As this happens, humanity as a whole will evolve. Our instinctual nature as a species will become more refined, more intelligent, and less fearful. Instinct will reveal its positive qualities, showing each individual the dimensions of creativity that exist within everyone.

Human emotions drive us to spiritual insight. You start to understand that spirituality is not outside you and that while its nature is unique to each person, there are common experiences that bind all people together. You will also learn that you do not need to be in a rush in order to know who you are and can be.

THE FIFTH FOUNDATION: ACCEPT THAT CONSCIOUSNESS IS IN EVERYONE AND EVERYTHING

We are an insecure species, each of us locked in our own little world. The quest for security can trick us in different ways. Our own worlds seem safe, whatever our personal circumstances. Even problems become a source of comfort, giving us a purpose and identity. From our small worlds we look out and judge others, but often, in our rush to evaluate them, we are misled by appearances. We see the outer shell but overlook the inner beauty in everyone and everything, the essence that contains liberating consciousness. Of course, it may be well hidden, but if we develop the sensitivity to perceive it, we find it is always there.

This awareness of a greater reality allows a transformative impulse to kick in. The desire for spiritual awakening can disrupt your existence in a major way. It comes from the innermost core of our humanity, where we are all aware of an inherent cosmic order. It allows us to move from an egocentric consciousness revolving around our intellect and emotions into a deeper universal consciousness, which leads us to a state of union with all life.

In this process, intellectual powers of reason, deduction, and creation change from a one-dimensional experience into multidimensional tools of time, space, and matter, emanating from the clear light of our highest being.

Each of us is a portal through which every aspect of energy within the universe may become aware of its own nature, a vibrant consciousness in search of itself. This energy, or frequency, is of such intensity that the universe can fashion itself as a human being or other animal, a plant, a rock, or a wad of chewing gum stuck to the pavement. But it is never divorced from itself; it remains its own center.

In this swirling cosmic consciousness, the day-to-day reality that you and I inhabit and the realities of our inner perceptions are always merged. This merging creates confusion: We must work within the sharp embrace of everyday reality but we also desire to experience pure universal energy. The confusion engenders a sense of separateness and a longing for meaning. We can, however, build a bridge between the two aspects of reality by infusing our desire for meaning with our sense of the nature of consciousness. We should not force this; simply becoming aware of the potential will help.

Benefits: Spiritual

In this aspect, you will start to unfold the higher dimensions of human consciousness, where you will experience the ways of integrating the everyday and the inner spiritual mind. The value of using spiritual insight in very practical ways—at work, say, or with your family, or to explore your creativity or simply to clean your windows better—becomes self-evident because it makes you sane and balanced. There is no benefit in experiencing higher aspects of human consciousness if it leaves you unbalanced. The higher you move within the aspects of your consciousness, the more you need to remember that. All spiritual experiences need strong foundations that can withstand the earthquakes of human consciousness as it moves toward a more profound recognition of itself.

Transforming the Five Senses

All of the five senses, which we take for granted on a daily basis, are pathways to making our souls. They underpin the physical, emotional, and mental structures that can enable us to find happiness, abundance, good fortune, health, and wisdom.

The senses are intimately connected to the mind. Most people think that the mind is comprised of thoughts and feelings, memories and sensations. In fact, these are the debris of the brain. The mind is the vast flowing expanse of high material energy that percolates through all things physical in this world and the universe.

The mind glues everything together, but through this very process it can ensnare itself, sandwiched between walls of desire and undeveloped consciousness. Our minds stay trapped much of the time, but transforming your senses and using their abilities and functions can safely remove the fortifications. Once liberated, your mind can connect with the larger mind energy of humanity.

We can learn to have direct experience of the spiritual universe by transforming our senses in a six-step process called Chilu. First, here is a short explanation of the potential of each sense, which you will see reflects the five foundations of the soul and their related benefits. When we experience our senses in a physical way, as most of us do, we have a limited sensory experience; but if we awaken them, through a special technique, which you will learn later, you will discover a particular type of consciousness for each sense and the color associated with it.

Sight

The sense of sight is about perception, looking into the heart of things, knowing your inner truth, and rediscovering your innocence and natural joyfulness. Transforming sight helps you to know what is behind your senses and what they are really for. Every sense is ruled by a color: For sight, this is a pure white light. The mental aspect of consciousness is awakened by this sense and color.

Smell

Through the sense of smell you learn about silence and also how all things are connected and interdependent. Forgiveness and the ability to love unconditionally are linked with smell. A warm and happy yellow light influences this sense. The emotional aspect of consciousness is awakened by this sense and color.

Hearing

Through your hearing, you can start to listen to your physical cycles and discover their wisdom and connections to inner energy. Hearing can help you to overcome fear and see through illusion. A blood-red light, warm, permeating, and life-giving, is linked to hearing. The intellectual aspect of consciousness is awakened by this sense and color.

Touch

Through your sense of touch, you will discover the nature of impermanence and that true success and happiness come about only by living in accordance with what makes you happy. The power to overcome obstructions is gained by training this sense. You will also learn about the value of wealth, money and power, and the nature of the material world. A gentle green light is associated with touch. The material aspect of consciousness is awakened by this sense and color.

Taste

The sense of taste enables you to experience how consciousness, spirituality, goodness, and happiness exist in everything, regardless of appearances or circumstances. A sky-blue light is connected with the sense of taste. The spiritual aspect of consciousness is awakened by this sense and color.

The Mind Tree

The transformation of your senses is manifest in the creation of a network of energy pathways that lead from the senses through the body to the brain and allow you to experience the spiritual universe more directly. The ancient Tibetans called this the "mind tree." The roots are in the brain, and its branches, leaves, fruits, and flowers are the five senses as they undergo the steps of transformation.

STEP 1
Sight

Sit comfortably with your eyes open. Instead of looking out through your eyes at the world, think that the world is flowing in through your eyes, gathering at the roof of your mouth, and then flowing down into the center of your chest. As the world flows through you it changes slowly into a flow of pure, sparkling white light. In your chest, it forms naturally into a sphere of vision and white light.

Smell

Sit comfortably with your eyes closed and place your attention inside your nose. Feel your nose smelling. Let whatever you smell gather at the roof of your mouth, then flow down into the center of your chest. As the smells flow through your body they transform into a beautiful yellow light. In your chest, it forms into a sphere of smell and yellow light, placing itself under the white sphere.

Hearing

Sit comfortably with your eyes closed and listen to all the sounds around you. Think of them flowing through your ears, into the roof of your mouth, gathering there, then flowing down into the center of your chest. As these sounds move within you, they become a beautiful blood-red light flowing through you into your chest. There it gathers itself into a sphere of all that you have heard and the beautiful red light places itself under the yellow sphere.

Touch

Sit comfortably with your eyes closed, hands together, cupped. Focus your mind on your hands, then let your awareness expand into each of your fingertips. Once you feel this, touch the atmosphere around you; allow it to flow into your fingertips, up through your arms and neck and into the roof of your mouth, where it gathers before flowing down into the center of your chest. All that you touch in the atmosphere turns into a green light flowing from the atmosphere into you. In your chest, this forms into a sphere and places itself under the blood-red sphere.

Taste

Sit comfortably with your eyes closed and your mouth gently open. Place all your attention on your tongue. Let the atmosphere and environment around you flow into it. Allow all of your body to flow into your taste buds. Let your body and the taste of the atmosphere and environment mix together where they gather at the roof of your mouth, and flow down into the center of your chest. As they flow down they become a sky-blue light, and form a sphere of tastes and sky-blue light that places itself under the green sphere.

You should have a line of spheres with the colors in this order radiating with their own special brilliance:

- White
- Yellow
- Blood red
- Green
- Sky blue

When you have the spheres in order, start to breathe in and out slowly through your nose. As you do this, each of the spheres becomes sealed within you.

Practice step 1 for a few minutes daily for three weeks. Then you can go on to the second step.

STEP 2

The practice is the same as in stage 1, but when the colored spheres are placed in order you do the following:

Working from the center of your chest, put the white sphere to your top left, the yellow sphere to your top right, the blood-red sphere to your bottom left, the green sphere to your bottom right, and the sky-blue sphere in the center, like this:

	White		*Yellow*
		Sky blue	
	Blood red		*Green*

Then, mentally direct the white light to the yellow sphere, the yellow to the green sphere, the green to the blood-red sphere, and the blood-red to the white sphere.

Next, direct light from the white sphere into the center of the sky-blue sphere. Do the same with the yellow, the green, and the blood-red spheres so that they are all connected. Take as long as you wish on this step.

Steps 1 and 2 will begin to increase the acuteness of your senses: You will physically see, hear, touch, smell, and taste more. Your overall health will improve as well as your everyday life. Often, physical illnesses or continuing psychological problems can improve and are sometimes cured by this practice.

STEP 3

Focus on the sky-blue sphere and let it become one with your physical heart. Imagine a channel of sky-blue light moving from the combined sphere and heart slowly up into the back of your neck and head, then up to the center of the top of your head. Then start to inhale from your heart to the top of your head; exhale from the top of your head out through your heart. Repeat step 2.

STEP 4

In this step you are going to breathe in all the colors of the spheres at once, taking them up the channel from the heart, through the neck and the back of the head to the center of your head. As you breathe in, draw them up gently without force. The colors will start to become intertwined like a rope of white, yellow, blood-red, green, and sky-blue strands. As you exhale from the top of your head and out through your heart, the colors return to their appropriate spheres. Do this for some time until you feel ready to move on to step 5.

STEP 5

Practice step 4 up to the point where the colored rope comes up to the top of your head. Then visualize all the colors cascading their brilliance over you, slowly and gently, like a waterfall of colors.

Your mind and body are awash with the flux and flow of these colors. Slowly, gently the movement subsides, and the rope of intertwined colors hangs in space above your head. Breathe in and out gently through your nose. The colored rope pulses with each inhalation and exhalation. At this point, imagine the rope transforming into an egg formed of all the intertwined colors, pulsing with beautiful light and the qualities of all your senses.

Gently and softly, but purposefully, sing the following sacred sounds. Each sound relates to a color that influences one of your senses.

*Sing a long A, so that the first sound is AAAAH, the second
LARRRM.*
AH: white light flashes within the egg (sight)
LAM: yellow light flashes within the egg (smell)
BAM: blood-red light flashes within the egg (hearing)
RAM: green light flashes within the egg (touch)
YAM: sky-blue light flashes within the egg (taste)

Wonderful feelings of purity and energy flow through your
mind and body. You feel refreshed, strong, and peaceful.

As you practice the steps, you will find that the entire
process becomes effortless and pleasant. Then you can move
on to the final stage, step 6.

STEP 6

In this step you can start to harmonize and integrate your
emotional, intellectual, physical, and spiritual worlds by activating the lights and the egg. Simply go on doing the steps and
send your thoughts to the light: They will create harmony in
anything you do.

After a while you will find that you can leave the intertwined rope of colors and the egg permanently active above the
center of your head. The energy behind your thoughts, actions,
and emotions can be stored and empowered within the egg,
thus increasing the quality and energy of your personality. This
builds your soul.

The rope and the egg are indestructible as long as you have
vitality. If you become ill, draw this energetic device back down
into the spheres. This particular form of Chilu is safe, powerful, and very relevant in today's world. It will empower you,
bringing enhanced mental clarity and at the same time
expanding and integrating consciousness into all aspects of
your life. It heals stress and helps you to create stress-free

actions. More important, it is a spiritual device that will bring happiness as you create deeper harmony in yourself. It can be used to help people overcome their fears of living as well as death and as a means to die well.

As you start to use this Chilu to develop your soul, do not strive to make it happen: Allow it to find its own time to grow and develop. Remember that you can do this, and experience the results, because within you is an innate goodness that seeks its way to full recognition and enlightenment. Your power, wisdom, and discernment have awakened, and, of course, your love for and of life, and your compassion for all that is. Remember, it is only compassion that can make all that is into all that it can be. Deep in the essence of all things is compassion.

Consciousness rejoices in itself, and this is compassion.

My senses pulsed with the light flowing through me. The world around me offered up new dimensions of awareness as my consciousness began to develop within the egg. I could feel and see this energetic rope of transformed senses flowing into the heart of the egg, and my soul began to be formed in front of me.

The higher aspects of my consciousness merged with the lower, the skillful with the clumsy, the refined with the rough. My humanity began to dawn upon me and its light was as vast as the planet.

All my senses had become pathways of intelligence, an intelligence born from the essence of my mind and the foundations of my consciousness. It was a self-creating intelligence, existing in everything, everywhere.

I had not become perfect, enlightened, or special. I had become more human.

Slowly I opened my eyes, breathed in the morning air, and looked at the fire smoking gently. I gazed at the mountain, the valley, and the lake. I gazed at my teacher and felt profoundly normal.

"Tea?" he asked, offering me a cup. I took the cup, absorbing its fragrance. As I brought it to my lips and drank, the tea and I drank each other.

Fusion.

CHAPTER THREE

Karma Mechanics

Tibetan medicine teaches that illness is a language that communicates the interacting forces of the mind and body. This language is common throughout the world, but many of us have forgotten what the "words" mean. We can no longer understand our own illnesses, or those of others.

Tibetan physicians are taught that human beings are always ill in some way, no matter how we appear. This is because our lives on this planet are effectively the working out of karma. Karma is the thread of invisible, intangible, all-pervading energy of which material life is woven. Karma is inescapable. It affects every living being all the time.

Enlightenment is the pure perfection that flows through moment to moment, millisecond to millisecond, in a continuous present where past and future are irrelevant concepts. Enlightenment is distinguished by the complete absence of egotism.

Compare that to our lives in this material world, where the past and present jostle to occupy the moment—where even the simplest action is complex, contingent on something or someone else. This is usually brought about by our perceived need to protect and promote ourselves.

Karma is the origin of all causes and conditions that shape our lives in this material world. From a Tibetan perspective, every event in our lives, big or little, creates another. It is these patterns that sow the seeds of further karma. Life well lived is a process of understanding this principle.

Karma is not romantic or spiritual, nor does it belong to special people. It is the stuff of birth and death, suffering and health—indeed, of all physical life, both active and dormant. Our characters and desires evolve from our past actions and thoughts. How and what we think; what we do and don't do; good thoughts, deeds, and habits, or bad ones; the way we see the world: "I'm bored with everything," "I hate my life," or the old favorite "It's all your fault"—all of these are responses and reactions to karmic influences.

One woman likens the concept of karma to a vast cosmic jigsaw puzzle:

> *For five decades, my life had been up and down, good and bad, simple and complex. It was like a vast jigsaw puzzle but no one had given me the box with the picture on it. I could see thousands and millions of tiny pieces tumbling and wheeling. Sometimes a few would come down and seemingly become organized, then the chaos would begin again. My life seemed happy but underneath it all, I had a suspicion everything might be pointless, including me. Taking the notion of karma on board gave me this most profound feeling that there is a big picture of my life, even though I may never see it.*

Karma is the key to understanding why we become ill, and illness itself is a direct way of understanding the karma we are experiencing. Why? Because illness can show us our emotional and physical patterns and the nature of personality and life-style—all of which are the functions of karma. Like all true healers and physicians, Tibetan doctors treat karma and its manifestations in the form of emotional and physical illness.

By understanding our karma, we come to know that everything changes, and this shows us how precious earthly life can be, for our lives are the one dimension of consciousness in which we can understand the nature of our karma.

A common misconception is that we are powerless to change the patterns of our lives. In fact, every little thing that helps us to be more conscious enables us slowly to improve the quality of our karmic energy. According to Tibetan teachings, every one of us has the potential to be enlightened, like the Buddha, and so to live a karma-free life. We may not get there this lifetime but we can start the process of creating good karma now. When you begin to accept the concept of karma, the first stirrings of awareness—however it appears to you—are delightful, thrilling, even mind-blowing. When you treat every person and every event in your life as a gift to help you on your spiritual journey, the way you perceive your life changes.

You begin to see the purpose. You feel connected.

The Attitude of Illness

Illness arises from an attitude deep within us, conditioning how we react to all kinds of suffering. This attitude comes from how we see ourselves in this world and the type of lessons that we have to learn. We often say how unfair it is when someone sweet and kind gets a fatal disease, or when young children get ill. How can such innocent beings be allowed to suffer?

The reason why we become ill is that our underlying attitudes are dealing with the lessons we need to learn as a result of past actions and thoughts.

Everyone on this planet is working out some karmic process of cause and effect. What we call illness is the result of a karmic attitude taking control of the body or the mind. Even great spiritual leaders are in the thrall of very subtle attitudes that cause them sickness or other forms of suffering. Other people's interactions can affect your karma, and yours can affect theirs. For example, His Holiness the Dalai Lama and all the great Buddhist and Bön teachers have suffered terribly due to the invasion of Tibet by the Chinese. According to many masters in different Tibetan traditions, this was prophesied many centuries ago and was caused by profound karmic interactions between China and Tibet.

Once these attitudes are in full swing, it can be difficult to change the mental process, particularly if the illness is serious and the body is deeply weak and unable to function. When the vital dynamics of the physical body lose strength, the mind may separate from the body. According to Tibetan medicine, this occurs when these attitudes have poisoned the vitality of the body-mind connection. The body grieves at the loss of the mind, and the mind panics with no body to carry its messages into the material world. The result is confusion. The vicious cycle continues as this confusion traps the illness, compressing it into sensations of unhappiness and fatigue and preventing any transformation into positive energy and recovery.

This problem arises when people cannot discern that the world is made up of interconnecting energies: mental, physical, and spiritual. These are the underlying and contributing energies known as the three humors, Wind, Bile, and Phlegm, which we will explore in later chapters. For now it is enough to say that the more separate a person's view of the world, the more strongly the karmic influence is expressed in illness.

Illness is here to help us stay connected to the ordinary events of life, and to remind us of our spiritual, emotional, and physical needs. We become ill because we forget our place in the natural cycle. The further we are removed from the concept of illness, the more likely we are to become ill. But, if we grow in self-knowledge and take responsibility for our thoughts and actions, we will slowly become aware of *why* we suffer and become ill.

Death, Rebirth, and Reincarnation

Karma is being created and worked out from moment to moment, day to day, and life to life. When people die they do not disappear, they change form. They then go through a rebirth, which is comparatively better or worse than the life they just left.

First of all, let us clear up the confusion between reincarnation and rebirth. Many people today talk about how problems, events, illness, or success come to them because of experiences from past lives. They talk about reincarnation and rebirth as if they are the same. But there is a big difference. When we die, the majority of us go through the process of dying with all the worries and confusions we carried in life. Because this stops us from being clear-minded in the death state, our next life happens without us directly choosing it. And the next, and the next, and so on. This is rebirth. We are endlessly cycled through existence by our own desires and karma.

Rare individuals, however, are able to choose the time, place, duration, and nature of their lives. That is reincarnation—the process of highly developed consciousness choosing where it goes. Such people could also, if they decided, choose not to be born again. For most of us, the most important life is the one we lead now—the years we have lived since we were

57

born this time. Studying the nature of this present life gives us insight about how to live in the future.

KARMA AND THE BIRTH PROCESS

So how do we become reborn? Well, it's a mixture of luck, timing, mental attitude, and karma. There is no shortage of wombs, but there is a shortage of good lives into which we can be born. Imagine you are bouncing around in the *bardo*, the state that we enter between death, birth, and life. Your consciousness craves a physical outlet, and, driven by karmic energy, you are drawn closer to your next parents as they make love. With a wallop and a bang, your gender is decided. Powerful emotions drive you to be a boy attracted to your mother, or a girl drawn to the father. You conceive a forceful dislike for the other parent at the moment of conception. Subtle karmic forces are set up for the rest of your life. Because of this, it can be easy for an individual to act out behavior that was relevant only to conception and time spent in the womb.

Pregnancy

Toward the end of pregnancy, your mother's womb feels like a solitary confinement cell in the worst prison imaginable. The baby form you inhabit experiences depression, anger, lust, and greed; it also feels toxic and polluted because the womb is full of poisons. The actual moment of birth is no better, because the birth process is similar to being beaten, or feeling that you are being burned alive.

The nature and length of the birth process is conditioned by your incoming karma, and how it interacts with the karma of your parents. Sometimes this is beneficial in that it creates good family relationships; other times it will create clumsy family relationships. All of this creates long-term psychological conditioning of your emerging personality.

HARD TIMES

Karmic events in our lives normally go in patterns of threes or fours, with each situation rapidly following the last. If you are experiencing a succession of problems of such intensity and significance that they cause you anxiety or despair, or reduce you to feeling that you have no control over your life, the underlying cause is karma working itself out. It may also be that these are life-changing events from which you can learn so that your life will get better—though maybe not immediately. Remember that karma is not a force against us; we have created it through our own thoughts and actions, informed by what we believed to be true at the time.

Creating Good Karma

Becoming aware of karmic processes, and deciding to change our karma for the better, is a profound shift that involves no action—merely a different perception that leads us gently into different ways of being and thinking and doing. As we understand these principles of karma, we reveal to ourselves the underlying flow of compassion, which is the bedrock of happiness and contentment. But as we uncover this compassion—exposing it in public—our everyday minds often go into a state of shock or even rebellion.

This happens because the more underlying self-knowledge we allow ourselves to see, the more the mundane habits of our lives become unglued. Our everyday minds are addicted to the comfort of their familiar routines, so, when they sense a threat, they throw up all sorts of land mines and smoke screens to prevent us from delving further.

If we forge on, we see that although many of our routines are valuable and sensible, they can restrict our lives and put brakes on our spiritual journeys. We can, however, transform the energy we put into everyday activities in simple ways. However humble and commonplace they are, each becomes a window through which we can see the divine. Like a baby chick cracking open the egg, that is the awakening of our own inner enlightenment.

An American patient came to me deeply unhappy. Financially he was well off, but mentally he had entered into a cold and isolated state. He told me that he was a drug dealer. I suggested that this line of work causes suffering to others and to himself.

After we had discussed it, he decided to return all his drug-dealing money to the communities that he had affected. In a Bön ritual of purification, he burned all the rest of his money, dollar by dollar; as he did so, he went through extreme psychic and physical pain. This process allowed him to start to burn off his self-made pollution.

He later turned himself in to the police and served time in prison. One of the drug squad that he confessed to is now a close friend. On his release he started a successful new business, which funds a nationwide nonprofit drug-rehab program that he set up.

This man found a spiritual path and also a loving wife. He turned his karma around by taking responsibility for his actions.

Generosity Heals All Things

Generosity is the first step on the path to improving your karma. This combination of emotional and intellectual energy is the single force that will help to burn away negative karmic patterns that may stop us from having the lives we want. Generosity heals all things and is part of the natural goodness that exists within us all.

Generosity is not just giving things to other people for their benefit. Primarily, it is giving with compassion and humor so that as well as benefiting the recipient, the energy of your generosity empowers them. They feel good in receiving what you offer. This attracts good fortune to them and thus radiates generosity into the world. Like the common cold, generosity can be easily caught and spread. It is a naturally spontaneous action, but it can also be planned and directed so that it becomes a skill that expresses our natural goodness.

Religion and philosophy often cause a greater lack of generosity than any other human activities. They are nothing more than buckets in which to carry refreshments for our souls to snack on. If you truly wish to experience an energy that can transform suffering and heal deep-seated karmic patterns for yourself and others, you must know that within all life there exists only one true teaching: love and kindness. There is nothing else.

GENEROSITY AND EQUALITY

The world may talk about equality, but, in fact, all living creatures are born unequal, because the machinery of power uses inequality as its fuel. Some people are more unequal than others. Equality will come about only as the karmic patterns on this planet lose their grip and transmute into new ways of interacting. Generosity of spirit, mind, and action is the first step in enabling all living creatures to become equal because implicit within true generosity is compassion. Every little kindness you do is a powerful step toward the gradual equality of all life on earth.

How to Develop Generous Energy

Be generous in the way your heart tells you to be. Never be generous merely because you think you should be. This is an unskillful mental action that will create clumsy events in the world around you and complicate your karmic patterns. Do not expect generosity to be returned. If you do, it becomes a business transaction, and you start to develop the habit of measuring value and worth. This diminishes your emotions, life force, and consciousness and creates further confusing karmic situations.

Results of Living Generously

When you are truly generous, the material energies of karma often create a process whereby life offers up a thank-you in the form of material benefit. But do not go looking for it, or life may slap you in the face. Generosity not only destroys negativities concerning work and financial success but helps to liberate you from inner fears and emotional conflicts of any type. Generosity creates thankfulness, so you start to live your life as a blessing. Being thankful for what you have is an act of generosity toward yourself.

This gratitude teaches you to become less attached to what you have and who you are. Paradoxically, this means that you value your material world more, because you are creating more emotional space that will be filled by positive energy. You are also free to love more widely and sincerely because you will be less attached to creating situations in which you hope to receive love from particular people.

As we work through our karma, we begin to understand that such love and kindness are simple and pure. It is often difficult to comprehend this. Karma can twist itself around love and kindness like a pretty, scented weed, shooting off in many directions. There are many good things about this weed; not least, that it heals us from doubt and fear. But eventually we must let it die and be reborn as a simple, unshowy healing herb.

By understanding the shifting patterns of karma in this way—from weed to herb—we can help to heal ourselves and find happiness, which are part of the natural cycle of our consciousness. And being happy helps us to recognize that life is essentially a spiritual experience.

A Single Thought Can Change Your Life Forever

Thinking is a skill that leads to self-knowledge. Self-knowledge is wisdom that is available to each and every one of us. Wisdom activates your consciousness. So, thinking well is good medicine. Most of the time, however, we don't think with the intention of creating an event or a situation that can enhance our lives: We think only in reaction to what has happened to us. One powerful way to create positive thoughts that support you to have a happy life is to improve the way in which you think, speak, and act.

For example, if you work for many years, months, or even days in a job you really hate, it will cause you to create negative behavior due to the negative emotions and thought patterns that build up within you. This creates a psychic pressure that hurts your emotional stability and diminishes your sense of well-being.

Harvey had worked for many years as a stockbroker. Since childhood he had experienced a great sense of loneliness. He thought that by making money he would feel safe and comfortable, and defend himself against loneliness.

After decades of incredible success, his work environment became intolerable. Harvey then did something that all his colleagues dreamed of but lacked the courage to do: He set up his own company. The economy was unhealthy and everyone said he would fail. In fact, he succeeded beyond his wildest dreams. But within a short time Harvey began to feel as he had before: unhappy, unfulfilled, and under pressure.

One day he woke up realizing that all of his working life had been a nightmare. He really hated his job, and working for himself intensified this experience. He lost interest. Slowly, his colleagues conspired to get rid of him.

When they succeeded in removing Harvey from his own company, he realized deep inside that he just didn't care. He started growing and selling organic apples and flowers. He made his own honey and discovered his inner happiness. He realized how the single thought of making money had caused him anxiety throughout his life. When he gave up this thought, he became happy.

This is just one example of the way in which millions of people all over the world unknowingly create negative or obstructional karma. Even when financial pressure is the root cause of the situation, we can look within ourselves to find answers to change the circumstances.

How to Think Better

Thoughts are the starting point both for words and for actions. Our world is ruled by the energy of thought, but it is not until we learn to think in a creative and responsible way that we can understand this truth. Remember: *According to Tibetan teaching, a thought—skillful or unskillful—is a fully developed situation that has yet to happen.* It is in this situation of potentiality that the karmic process is ready to move from a dormant state into an active force, bringing what we regard as good or bad situations.

Some of these situations are dramatic highs and lows, but most of the time our karma simply brings a continual flow of experiences, routines, and habits. Although they may appear to be mundane, they are of great spiritual importance. To understand our karmic influences, both on ourselves and on other people, we need to know more about the energy of our thoughts and those of others. Unskillful thoughts attract negative energy, which in turn creates unskillful events, actions, and outcomes. Clear and skillful thinking, however, brings harmony, contentment, and peace.

You need first to understand and then to analyze the kind of thinking patterns you formed in the past. There are five types of unskillful thinking patterns that can chatter simultaneously in our minds. These can be seen in every culture across the ages. If you consider that they are the basis of the way most people conduct their lives, it's easy to see why society is ill. Unskillful thinking pollutes the mind, which in turn pollutes the world. All of these thinking patterns can create good or bad results; the key is to learn what they have to teach you.

Unskillful Thinking Patterns

1. Thinking patterns that make you unrealistically optimistic:

    Optimism is a natural impulse in thinking. Over-optimism is an energy that is not refined or balanced. Overly optimistic people are prone to creating fantasies that they know will not come true, rather than realistic blueprints from which to work. Although they genuinely like others, people who think this way often feel essentially lonely. The more you fall into thinking patterns that make you overly optimistic, the more disconnected you become from your emotions. If it is not harmonized, this impulse can cause emotional exhaustion. From a Tibetan medical view, it can also lead to a growing state of inner panic and anxiety that can contribute to the thinker's susceptibility to cancers of the throat, lungs, or thyroid. Lower-back conditions, migraines, and phobic cycles also come from this state.

A good thinker is an architect of consciousness. Skillful thinking is the process of assembling energy and constructing an edifice that makes ideas or events real. If we can become skillful thinkers, there will be social, cultural, and global change of huge importance. Individuals will start to become more responsible for their actions. We will understand the need for mutual cooperation. We will feel the impact of thought as it occurs, and the world will become linked by an empathic connection that will help to bring greater social integration to all societies. We will be at the beginning of understanding one another.

2. Thinking patterns that lead you to be fearful, gloomy, and depressed:

Virtually all of us feel afraid and low at some point in our lives. However, Tibetan medicine says that when someone's thinking patterns start to involve these mental states on a regular or daily basis, the mind is reacting to karmic forces created because the individual has been overwhelmed by the world around him or her.

Normally, people who experience these states live in fear of communicating with other people. The concept of shyness covers this experience to a degree, but at the heart of this fear is really a deep sense of isolation and abandonment. If this state is not healed, the person may become susceptible to addictive behaviors, mental illness, skin conditions, and problems with the central nervous system in later life.

3. Thinking patterns that cause you to focus solely on material outcomes such as money, career, and relationships:

Focusing your attention completely on having possessions and controlling people, resources, and events eventually becomes the equivalent of committing a slow suicide. People who do this have forgotten how to live. They have become divorced from life. Sadly, there are millions living like this globally, creating social unrest and a slow rotting of social integrity, which exerts an unseen pressure on others to conform.

You may say that it's understandable, even admirable, for poor people to think obsessively about money and work. But it actually decreases their opportunities for advancement because their obsessive thinking starts to build up within them, creating mental piles of rubbish. The more narrowly we focus, the more opportunities we lose for change. We risk becoming caught up in acting out the obsession and not achieving the goal.

People who focus on relationships do so because they hope that those on whom they are focusing will enable them to gain control of their own situations. Equally, people who make themselves the center of attention are using others as buffers to defend themselves against the imagined harshness of their lives.

When wealthy people have tunnel vision about work and money, it stems from a lack of faith in their achievements: They feel that fundamentally they have no value. I know a billionaire who is trapped by the world he has made. He has no faith in what he has achieved, yet he feels he must organize everything so that it can continue. He sleeps little, dresses humbly, and drives a small car, not because he wishes to be anonymous but because he has no sense of value about his wealth or achievements. He is scared of people and he is starting to find out why.

Sometimes a peson will focus exclusively on an intense relationship with one special person or a group of people. This is because the individual wants to like and approve of himself. The people he looks at serve as mirrors, reflecting the image that the individual wants to see and believe in.

These types of people are susceptible to arthritis, rheumatism, gout, Parkinson's disease, Steele's syndrome, and a wide range of other inflammatory and nervous system disorders. Cancers of the gall bladder, liver, and bowel are also common.

4. Thinking patterns that lead you to obsess about physical and sexual activities:

When people dwell only on these matters, it is because they are emotionally and spiritually stuck; it is not because they seek greater emotional intimacy. They do so because unconsciously they feel that they have lost connection to the spiritual energies of their personalities and to the world around them. So, they focus on physical or sexual activities to increase vitality and energy and to feel connected and alive.

Illness of the musculoskeletal system is common to these types of thinkers, as are sudden bouts of depression. Most experience great loneliness in later life.

5. Thinking patterns that make you focus on spiritual, artistic, or religious activities, while denying the material world, your own culture, and its influence on you:

This type of thinking pattern takes place when a person is consumed with the search for truth and meaning but is pursuing it in an unskillful and unproductive manner. Spiritual transformation, artistic endeavor, or religious vocation of any lasting value comes through some form of interaction with one's culture, material realities, and art. These are the catalysts and mediums through which constructive and liberating thinking patterns take place in this life.

This type of thinker is susceptible to addictions of any type, mental illness, all forms of cancer, dental diseases, and conditions affecting the reproductive organs and the eyes. These people also tend to dislike humanity, disregard authority, and be culturally intolerant.

The more you know about negative thinking patterns, the more you will be able to engage in constructive thinking. Simply being aware of them allows you to start clearing your mind of these untamed thoughts and the emotional pain they create. You can do this by looking deeply within yourself for a few minutes every day and reflecting on whether any or all negative thoughts are moving within you. Surprisingly quickly, you will gain insight into how such thought processes affect you personally, and also how you affect other people and the world around you. This in turn reduces the general karmic fallout in your life.

As your mental and spiritual energies become stronger, the general level of your thinking becomes more powerful, as does the quality of your emotional experiences. The process of weaving your own karma will also become profound, effortlessly. You will find yourself imbued with a deeper sense of responsibility for the way you think and behave toward yourself and all other living creatures. If you decide to accept this responsibility, you will begin to understand that all living things seek to communicate.

What they want to communicate is wisdom, happiness, and the unconditional compassion that flows through us all and that is our foundation as living creatures.

CHAPTER FOUR

Awaken the Wisdom Within

Each of us has an infinite capacity for wisdom. However, we must choose to connect with it. Wisdom is not a beginning or an end in itself, it is the process by which we can transform our physical and emotional worlds. It changes and adapts itself to the forces and circumstances around it. The goal is to discover and liberate our consciousness so that each of us can discover the divine in everything and, through that, joy and the immeasurable possibilities of life.

Wisdom comes in many forms, but its underlying essence is the force, or energy, that holds the material and the natural worlds together. It is in every living thing on this planet, regardless of appearance. It is the song of nature; it has rhythms, pulses, and beats. Listening to the rhythms of wisdom enables you to become connected to the life force of the planet. Connecting with wisdom enables you to use the energy of thoughts and actions skillfully.

Many people are confused about the nature of wisdom because they see it as influence over other people. They confuse wisdom with its effect. According to the ancient Tibetans, true wisdom is wisdom over oneself. No one can rob you of your potential for wisdom. Nor do you need to wear it like a badge; it has no need to show itself unless it is needed.

There is no such thing as perfect wisdom or perfect knowledge about wisdom. It is entwined in the essence of each human being, so it is just as variable as we are. It does not need to be forced, merely understood. Then it naturally enables you.

Connecting with wisdom comes through winning the battle of the heart. This is the war between emotion and intellect, right and wrong, good and bad. It is won when you know the nature of your personality. True wisdom manifests itself in your relationships with other people, and one of its great qualities is that it enables you to behave with compassion, humility, and good humor in all things.

The starting place is simple, although the path may be difficult. You need to be prepared to be full of love. This means learning to accept all the hardships and obstructions in your life so that you can begin to strip away the emotional junk that we all carry.

When consciousness is stuck in matter, as it is in this incarnation, we can become seduced into believing that the material things that enthrall our senses are valid and necessary. Inner wisdom helps us to cast out addictions to glamour, gurus, and everything else that takes us away from who we really are and can be.

The exercising of wisdom is a natural process that is constantly available to those who are prepared to look beyond the appearances of the everyday world. People are afraid of looking for wisdom because they do not want to look too closely at themselves. But if you are able to live with yourself in this way—opening the windows of your perception to look beyond the routine, superficial, and mundane—life responds to you with open arms and an open heart.

We can experience this quite simply by not entering into a state of judgment about people, situations, and events. Just accept them as they are, without criticism or comment. Instead of being judgmental, be discerning. Being judgmental is unskillful emotional behavior because you color a person, situation, or event with your own prejudice. Being discerning means trying to be open at all times, to allow knowledge to come to you naturally. Be, think, and do what feels right. Feel the energy in this approach. All things will reveal themselves to you if your heart is open.

To those who know how to ask, the world seeks to give all that they want. To those who are one with their wisdom, the skill of asking and the gift of receiving come naturally. Tasting the sweetness of your inner wisdom releases many answers to the questions that you have about life and the issues that are important to you. Although, paradoxically, you may often not really know the question until you have received the answer. Then you suddenly realize that it was something that had been bothering you for ages.

The issues can be about anything or anyone—trusting that an important favor had been carried out by a friend, for instance, or that a job you had paid for was completed. Nagging doubts about anything—from the unimportant to the crucial in the past, present, or future—are resolved through information and circumstances coming together.

Being connected to wisdom does not mean that your life will be free of problems or difficulties. But you will know how to solve, transform, and release them so that they will not repeat themselves. There are many benefits. This wisdom in our daily lives acts as a stabilizer and a healing force and will often show us the direction we should take in life. Also, acting wisely in our everyday lives energizes the people around us.

As you connect with your wisdom, you will discover the meaning of an ancient Tibetan principle: "All community comes from the community of one." This means that once you are united with your inner wisdom, there are no divisions or conflicts in your life. All material aspects of mind—intellect, emotions, and everyday living—flow from your consciousness in one coherent stream.

True wisdom sustains everything.

The Starting Point

It is the knowledge that our lives have meaning that enables us to experience both wisdom and pleasure. It is meaning that gives wisdom its value and ultimate use. If there were no point to our lives, why would we want or need wisdom?

Through the years there are signposts that offer us opportunities to understand the meaning of our lives. We can learn to recognize the special omens that will lead us to turning points.

We must start with an experience to which all human beings are attracted: beauty. Beauty is a doorway to wisdom and can be an expression of it. The ancient Tibetans believed that beauty can be a way to understand the nature of the material world because as material beauty fades, spiritual beauty grows. Connecting with our own inner beauty allows us to discover that we are sacred. This is what beauty is for, a display of sacredness in the material world.

By knowing the nature of inner and outer beauty, you can activate it within you and in your life.

How to Release Immense Wisdom: The Eight Material Activities

People in ancient Tibet were no different from people in today's world: They too had troubles, doubts, and fears. But nowadays, because of the pressures of modern living—commuting to work, stress, crime, unemployment, and all the other problems we live with daily—we cannot see how to ease our problems. The key is to know the energy at the core of the problems.

This is revealed by examining what the Tibetan Bön and Buddhist traditions call the "eight material activities." These describe the nature of our feelings. They are the mental building blocks that fuel all human endeavor and influence the way we respond to the events and people in our lives. They are: loss, shame, guilt, and suffering; and achievement, fame, approval, and happiness.

Whether seemingly negative (the first four) or positive (the second four), the material activities have immense power over our lives. We absorb these characteristics from childhood and then start to use them to define our everyday realities. They create confusion in our minds, handcuffing us to a desperate search for what we believe is happiness, and an equally intense desire to avoid unhappiness. You have only to look at your life and the lives of others to see how we are all affected.

The results of being attached to these feelings are unpredictable and often uncontrollable. Wisdom comes when we can see that the eight material activities are born from anger, lust, and greed. They urge people to create and to destroy. We may long for, say, approval, but in chasing it we damage others and expose ourselves to shame. We take an important job not because we really want to do the work but for the status and money it brings. We have a relationship with someone not because we truly love and empathize with them but because we bask in the security of their approval.

The wise action is to cut the cords of attachment to all the material activities, the positive as well as the negative, so that our lives are not defined by them. This makes us truly free.

To do this we must learn to accept all the aspects of our

personalities—the light and the dark—without judgment, and to understand that both happiness and unhappiness are good. Then we can receive and give thanks for the good times and for the bad.

True wisdom comes from the mind and creates its own freedom. Understanding the energy wielded by these material activities helps to eliminate their influence over you. You become able to use your energy, thoughts, and actions skillfully and appropriately. You surrender your fears and become more compassionate and patient. You will find that your life naturally starts to improve and good fortune begins to flow in.

The ancient Tibetans often described the way in which our emotions influence us as a turbulent mountain river. This is a traditional Bön story, which illustrates the different ways in which three people are conditioned by the eight material activities.

A man stood on the edge of a river. Although it was narrow, the current was strong. The angry water seemed a mirror image of his mind, throbbing and tossing with the eight material activities. He decided to let them flow out of his mind into the water. His mind became calm and his heart content.

Suddenly he heard a shout for help and in the white foam of the waves he saw a man from his village. He hated this man because he had had sex with his wife, stolen his livestock, and then beaten him at wrestling. Then another cry for help came to his ears. In the water he saw a very holy saint whom he respected greatly. He had helped him in times of trouble and had eased his mind.

Both men were being dragged to the edge of a dangerous waterfall. He knew they would be drowned. With great effort he hurled his hunting rope to the other side of the river. The noose tightened fast around a rock and he tied the other end to a tree.

Both men caught on to the rope and pulled themselves to safety. But once on the riverbank they began to fight. The holy man started screaming, "I tried to stop you from jumping in and you pulled me in with you. Now look at me! I'm soaking wet."

The other man just laughed hysterically and punched the holy man on the nose. "You do-gooders are all the same," he said. "I never asked you to help me."

At this, our brave hero became upset and confused, and his body tensed up. Then he suddenly realized that these men were not real but personifications of the eight material activities.

With a yell he pushed them back into the river and they plunged screaming over the waterfall, down into the seething water. He sat on the riverbank exhausted, the screaming still echoing in the rocky gorge around him.

But doubt sneaked into his mind like a thief. He started panicking about pushing the two men back into the waterfall. What if he was wrong . . . ?

This story illustrates the subtle pervasiveness of the eight material activities. Here is a man wanting to be at peace by ridding himself of the activities. As he lets them flow from his mind, he experiences the achievement of peace and contentment. But when he sees his enemy drowning, he feels shame, loss, guilt, suffering, and also happiness. Then he notices the holy man and experiences happiness and the lure of fame. When his enemy and the holy man start fighting, he goes through shame, loss, guilt, and suffering. Then he experiences the relief of recognizing that they must be an illusion created by the eight material activities. Peace again. He can push both men back into the river because they are not real. Then his everyday mind comes up with a new problem: Just suppose he was wrong?

How to Connect with Inner Wisdom by Living in the Space Between Moments

Memories glue our lives together. Memories are moments. Moments are frozen experiences, squeezed out of the eight material activities. Life is a series of these moments, which turn into the blur we call reality.

Many of us believe that we should try to live in the present moment, but this is unwise for two reasons. Our brains cannot experience reality directly because everything has to be received and interpreted through our senses. So we live in the past, always a few seconds behind. We can't experience the moment directly; it has passed before we can even comprehend it.

Furthermore, moments are entire worlds of experience, immense and complex. To live in the moment with our everyday minds would be almost impossible. It would risk making us nearly as frantic and busy, exhausted, and unconnected to the world around us as living in the past and the future make us.

The place to live is not in the moment but in the space between moments—a space that holds a continual flow of wisdom and consciousness. By connecting to the space between the moments of your life, you start to experience what is, not what was.

Wisdom is everywhere, waiting to be received and used. But we can understand wisdom only when we are at our most humble, and we can go beyond the moment, into the space between, only when we truly understand that the only thing separating the everyday world from the world of wisdom is a transparent curtain.

Think of a time in your life when you had nowhere and no one to turn to. In that state of being unable to cope, there is an inner dialogue taking place between your frightened everyday mind—which is made up of the eight material activities—and your inner wisdom, which consists of nothing but itself.

If, in those situations, you can enter the space between moments and rest in your wisdom, you will find that it will comfort your everyday mind, allay its fears, and allow it to start anew. You are all the wisdom you need.

How to Enter the Space Between Moments: A Meditation

Make yourself comfortable, sitting, lying down, or in a favorite meditation position. Close your eyes and look within yourself as far as you can see. You will sense an inner horizon. When you reach it, look beyond. When you can see no more, rest within yourself. This looking inward sometimes gives the sensation of traveling within yourself.

In this place of rest, listen to your inner world. Slowly you will hear the rumbling of your everyday mind: It may sound like a train, a storm, or a large crowd of people talking. Listen again and under the noise you will hear a slow and exquisite sound, like a soloist singing a beautiful song, a choir, the playing of a cello, or a distant wind. That is your inner wisdom.

Don't feel that you have to do anything with this wisdom when you find it. Just allow it to percolate naturally into your life. Be with it. You will find that simply knowing it's there— remembering the way it appeared to you, sensing its nature— will take you naturally into the space between moments and allow the experience to become second nature in your daily life.

You can do this meditation once a day for as long or short a time as you wish. Do not force or regiment it; you will find that a natural cycle develops and this will guide you.

Inner wisdom can change the outer world. Experiencing the space between moments may take just a second yet permeate your entire life, creating opportunities for dynamic change and healing. The sacred stillness that stays in your everyday mind is the fountainhead of the constant wisdom that flows through your life and the natural world. The way your mind works, how you view the world, and your feelings about life can be refreshed and restored.

USING THE EIGHT MATERIAL ACTIVITIES TO DIAGNOSE THE CAUSE OF YOUR INNER TROUBLES

Understanding the material activities and how they affect you can help you to create a balanced life. The following stories tell of two people who experienced every one of the activities and of how their lives suffered in consequence.

By using the meditation technique described above to tune in to the dialogue between their inner wisdom and their everyday minds, they were able to gain insight into how and why they had suffered. They understood how they created their problems, reacted to them, and then played them out in a continuing cycle.

This understanding empowered them to live more skillful lives and to create real happiness. Their stories highlight the way in which people can turn things around, if they choose to do so.

Like most of us, Laurent, a singer, and Bruce, a doctor, had allowed the eight material activities to become the foundations of their lives. From their perspectives at the time, they believed they had experienced them positively. In their different ways, both had star-spangled careers that brought them fame, status, and approval. Neither had experienced shame, loss, or guilt. Other people saw them as members of the "great and good" club. But then it all went wrong.

At age fifty-five, Laurent was at the peak of her career as a country-western singer in the United States. She seemed to have it all: constant success, huge amounts of money, and an adoring husband and family. She was loved and idolized around the world.

But inside, Laurent felt empty and shoddy, as if she were made of mud and straw. On tour, audiences noticed that she had lost her spark. Slowly her career dried up and she found herself at home in her mansion with nothing to do and nowhere to go.

Then one of Laurent's two daughters died in a plane crash. Later, the other was seriously injured in a car accident. Laurent started to drink too much. Her husband ran away with her best friend, taking a large amount of Laurent's money with them. Laurent's drinking escalated into alcoholism.

Completely lost, Laurent came to see me. As she began to recover from the pain of betrayal and her alcohol addiction, we discussed the eight material activities and how they had been expressed in her life. They gave her an insight into why her life had fallen to pieces.

"My whole life was based on one big false image and I believed it so much that I didn't allow myself to see that, deep inside, I knew the truth. My inner self was yelling at me to wake up but I couldn't hear—didn't want to hear— until it all came crashing down."

Laurent knew that each of the material activities had contributed to her obsessive drive for money and fame from an early age. Now she understood that they were covering up a spiritual need that had never been fulfilled. She realized that her old life had weak foundations and that her everyday mind functioned only by knee-jerk reactions—

conditioned by the material activities—to every event in her life. As her true personality eroded, her life fell to pieces, because the blueprint that she was following was flawed.

Today, Laurent has a new life with a different focus—her own happiness. Day by day, she is recovering from her alcoholism. No longer does she use her fame to gloss over her problems. She does the occasional concert, singing for joy rather than for money and status, and her musical career has recently taken off again. She hasn't met a new love, but she isn't worried. She feels connected to herself and to the world. She is content.

Bruce, a celebrated trauma specialist in the emergency room of a big hospital in the Deep South, saved lives daily. Quiet-mannered and soft-spoken, everyone looked up to him as a perfectionist who could always be relied on. Behind the calm facade, however, was a different story.

Bruce himself was traumatized by the suffering of his patients—victims of violent crimes or appalling accidents—and by a fear of failing in front of his colleagues. Driven by his own demons, he became more and more successful. He believed that his work made him happy until something within him began to fail. He made a wrong diagnosis, his patient died, and a court case followed where he was publicly humiliated.

The man who could do no wrong was now reviled by his community. There was no one to fight on his side, none of the approval on which he had depended for years. He broke down.

When Bruce came to see me, he told me that he had started to lose his spirit long before making the misdiagnosis. He was on burnout. Like Laurent, he was falling to pieces. His breakdown was the end of a long process.

As Bruce learned the meditation practice described above,

he started to realize how the eight material activities had conditioned his life. He felt he had become a walking, talking machine fueled by material aspirations—money, house, car, fame, sex—which were far from the reasons he'd originally gone into medicine. He had forgotten his desire to make sick people healthy and the world a better place.

As we talked, he remembered an inner conviction that he'd had from early on—that there is something inside human beings that influences our lives and our states of health; something that makes us sick or well. Curiously, it was something that he had buried during his career in medicine.

This realization was the beginning of his exploration into the relationship between his everyday mind and his inner wisdom. Along the way he found that despite his feelings of shame and guilt over his patient's death, he was a worthwhile person.

Today, Bruce is working again as a physician, but this time in a desert community, far from the bright lights and big-city environment he craved before. Rather than patch up broken bodies, he heals emotional and physical ills. He uses the eight material activities as one of his diagnostic tools, working with his patients to uncover their underlying problems.

Bruce says he feels happier now. He knows who he is and he wants to help other people to do the same.

Everyone has the power to awaken the wisdom within. We have only to try. All we have to lose is our unhappiness. Look inside. Listen to the dialogue between your everyday mind and your inner wisdom. They seek to communicate so that you may become whole, happy, and empowered.

Starting Over: Breathing a New Persona

The simplest and most basic way to start your new life is through breathing. We are what we breathe, and we are *because* we breathe. It is the spirit of life.

According to Tibetan wisdom, the universe is a living, breathing organism. Breath is the underlying psychic makeup of the material universe, connecting everything in the cosmos. So every breath we take links us to the inhalation and exhalation of the universe.

This connection through the nature of the breath is more than just physical; it is essential in creating our humanity and consciousness. Breathing gives us the ability to love, and the breathing patterns that we develop dictate our attitudes toward money, material achievement, and success and failure.

Tibetan wisdom states that although we breathe automatically, breathing is not an unconscious action. The problem is that through our unthinking, clumsy attitude, we have come to treat it as if it were. By learning to master the huge resource that exists within our breathing, all of us can reveal our potential. Deep in the process of respiration is practical wisdom that can be released to our conscious minds.

There are nine dimensions of breathing, each of which can empower an aspect of our personalities. Let us now explore each of these and how, together, they build the energetic architecture that creates the foundations of our personas. You will find a simple meditation with each dimension, which will help you to absorb it into your life. With this, you can use your breathing to inspire your life.

Choose a calm and peaceful environment for your meditation: Don't worry if the only place you can find is at your desk or on a bus—just do the best you can. Uncross your arms and legs, close your eyes, and relax. Breathe gently and rhythmically. In these meditations you will focus mainly on negative situations. Be sure not to judge yourself harshly. Just be loving to yourself and to the problem.

The Nine Dimensions of Breathing

1. Personality and Emotion

This first stage influences the way in which we interact with the world around us and the intensity of our emotions. It is in this stage that all our self-knowledge exists, waiting to be activated. Our first breath at birth sets the emotional nature of our personalities for the rest of our lives—unless and until we choose to change it. Because breathing sets up the personality, meditating on this first cycle can help you to reinvent your life.

MEDITATION

Reflect on whatever you are unhappy with in your personality and your emotions. Try to define what doesn't feel right and look at it without judging yourself. For instance, if you feel you have a problem with anger, or gossiping, or being negative, start off by saying to yourself: "I am aware that I get angry/gossipy/negative and of the effect that has on me and on other people."

Repeat this several times. Take a slow breath in, hold it for a few seconds, then breathe out slowly. This will help to purify and transform your anger or other negative characteristics.

You can do this simple meditation for any conflict you feel within you or for any personality trait that you want to transform. Do it for ten minutes, twice a day, for twenty-seven days.

2. Intellect

As the first stage creates our emotional reality, so the second creates our intellectual ability. The intensity, quality, and nature of the intellect is set up by this breathing cycle. This breathing pattern affects us all the time, as our intellectual abilities are constantly changing.

Your emotional energy dominates your intellect and all the other dimensions. However, your intellectual energy cannot change your emotions.

MEDITATION

If you find it hard to think clearly or to concentrate on an intellectual or academic discipline of any sort, you can stimulate the second dimension of your breath by focusing on a conflict or subject that is causing you a problem. Breathe in and out, focusing on the issue, then imagine that your intellect is a single flame flowing down into the power center in your navel. Breathe in the flame, hold it for a moment, then breathe it out, directing the fiery energy to your mind. This will purge your intellect, burning away the confusion.

3. Physical Health

This third breathing pattern directly influences your body's state of health. It is the one pattern of which most people are aware. When we become ill, our breathing always changes.

By understanding the nature of breathing in this cycle, you can have a direct and powerful influence over your health and physical well-being. By training your breath, you can learn how your body works and, if it's not working, how to repair it. Good health is actually good insight about your body; discovering this puts you in control.

Meditation

Whether you are currently feeling well or ill, you can practice this meditation to optimize your health. Start by breathing normally. If you are well, focus on your heartbeat and allow your inhalations and exhalations to align with it. If you are ill, take long, deep breaths, then hold your breath for as long as you comfortably can. Think about the illness and the symptoms. Identify the key words that describe your condition and say them to yourself while you breathe out slowly and gently. Do this five times, then again link your breath to your heartbeat.

4. Adaptability

The fourth stage in the breathing cycle that makes up our personalities becomes more dominant whenever mankind as a species is in a period of global change, because it gives us the ability to successfully adapt and change to circumstances and events. It also embodies our potential to create a profound connection with the forces of nature.

According to ancient Tibetan Bön teachings, it was this breathing cycle that dominated every part of human consciousness in the earliest times on earth—an era of vast change. As the species developed in Neolithic times, this particular aspect of the breathing cycle diminished. Only in the turbulent last five hundred years has this aspect of the breathing cycle returned to common consciousness in the everyday world.

Meditation

This will help if you have trouble in accepting change or find it hard to adapt to changing circumstances. Sit quietly and focus your mind on the situation and circumstances. As you do this, let the essence of the situation come to you: Sometimes it seems unlikely, but you will find that your instinct is always right. Hold this essential truth as your mantra and chant it aloud as you slowly breathe in and out. Do this once a day, for as long as you are able, for nine consecutive days.

5. Wealth and Abundance

This fifth stage relates to the nature of money, wealth, abundance, and resources. By cultivating this aspect of breathing, you start to attract a more harmonious flow of resources to you.

If you are prepared to share what you have, it is your right to have what you need—indeed, to have *more* than you need. If at the end of your life you have great wealth and do not share it, you create deep mental obstructions that diminish your happiness before you die.

Good fortune waits within the forces of your unconscious mind, so the world of money and abundance responds to this cycle of breathing. You must be ready for it, though, because it can have a more toxic effect on your mind and emotions than fame has. You will keep your good fortune only if your heart is also abundant with love and generosity.

MEDITATION

Sitting quietly with your eyes closed, breathe in and out. Clap your hands together as loudly as you can to purify the atmosphere around you. Focus on your breathing slowly for a few moments, then in your mind's eye see your inhalations drawing up wealth and abundance from within you. As you exhale, direct this abundance out into the world as raw energy. It will automatically come back to you, like a boomerang. To end the meditation, say quietly but firmly, out loud, "I thank the world, I thank all things, I thank my awakening good fortune." Clap your hands loudly and slowly three times, and, if you wish, bow to north, south, east, and west, and then to the ground beneath your feet.

6. Friendship

This cycle relates to our roles as friends and parents. According to Tibetan wisdom, a friend is a person who not only shares the important times in your life but can also act as a spiritual guide, bringing insight to your needs and dilemmas.

This dimension of breathing reveals how we see ourselves in the world. Our friends are reflections of ourselves. We have them because we need them.

When it comes to parents, the process becomes more acute. Our parents reflect our journey in life, showing us possible karmic experiences that need to be resolved. These karmic experiences are neither good nor bad, just a part of the process that people must go through to gain a more complete self-knowledge. Tuning in to this breathing cycle can help us fully comprehend the reasons why we chose the parents—and the children—that we did.

MEDITATION

This exercise helps us to connect with and care for other people. You can use it to heal problems with friends or family. Sitting silently, close your eyes and direct your attention to the person with whom you are in conflict. As you inhale, imagine that you are breathing this person into you. As you exhale, breathe out any negativity. You can do this with an individual, a group, or everyone on the planet. You simply visualize great crowds as your friends and family, using your breath to draw them into your heart and mind.

7. Integrity and Morality

In the seventh cycle, we discover the process of self-responsibility and the importance of developing integrity and a personal moral code. Morality cannot be taught but it can be experienced by understanding a little of your personality. It is within this cycle that self-empowerment takes place and the search for meaning in life is to be found.

The seventh cycle is profoundly affected by the sixth; the two are often deeply interwined within people's lives. The foundations, structures, and habits we have toward personal relationships are played out in this cycle. The sixth cycle can profoundly influence a person's search for love, and the seventh is linked to intimate personal relationships.

It is here, also, that the differences between men and women are created on the energetic level. This energy is not just physical and psychological but becomes, for both genders, a special and different experience of the planet.

MEDITATION

Within everyone there exists pure integrity and a deep moral awareness. This exercise will help you to connect with these qualities of your inner nature and experience them in your daily life. Sitting in silence with your eyes closed, focus on your heartbeat. As you breathe, see your breath creating a light within your physical heart. Pink at first, it glows more powerfully with each breath until it radiates a pure white incandescence that spreads purity and integrity throughout your body and mind. Merge with this white light, and the true nature of your inner morality will be clear to you.

8. Trust

This cycle of breathing has a profound association with the experience of trust and safety. Ultimately this has to do with trusting the natural order of life and feeling safe with oneself and with other people in the greater play of life and its circumstances.

The eighth breathing pattern teaches us that all things will ultimately be harmonious; that there is a meaning to the sometimes overwhelming chaos that is casually termed *life*. Life is not bigger than you or me, but the events of life can seem that

way. We have to realize that those events are not life, just inci-
dents that mark the passage of life through your experience of
living. You are life, as we all are.

MEDITATION

In order to trust other people and the world around us, we
need to connect with the earth. We are children of the earth
and dependent on it for all material things; this connection is
the bedrock of any form of trust. Find a pebble or handful of
soil and sit comfortably, with your eyes closed, holding it. As
you breathe in, imagine its energy flowing into you and connecting you directly with the earth. The pebble or soil is nothing except what it is, and that is the nature of pure trust. Do
this exercise once a day when you wake up.

9. Life, Death, Rebirth

The last of the nine cycles of breathing reveals to us that all
things are renewed. It is one of the great beauties of the universe, that all things continue regardless of death or any other
kind of ending, whether they take the form of people, rocks,
buses, or teacups. Death simply means a change of energy and
form.

The ninth cycle holds within it the very impulses of life
energy. It shadows the other eight, often coming to us in times
of introspection or in dreams. It is most active when we are
born, again when we have our first sexual experiences, and
when we are about to die. It is the essence of the evolution of
our species.

MEDITATION

With your eyes closed, breathe slowly. See each inhalation and
exhalation as a stream of light carrying you deep into the
underlying essence of everything, where you can sense the
energetic foundations of the universe. As you breathe, let your-

self be absorbed into this clear, sparkling light until you fuse with the light. You are the light and it is you.

Practice this meditation once a week, building up to one hour, if possible. You will begin to experience the interconnection of all the nine dimensions.

"Your breath is the only thing that you own," my teacher told me.

Through these meditations you may see that it is the only thing that you need.

CHAPTER FIVE

Emotional Healing

Our emotions are the origins of our physical health. The emotional dynamics within us set up patterns that are then implemented in our body, where in time they become patterns of well-being or of poor health. In order to be truly healthy it is vital to understand and balance the emotional dynamics within us.

Few of us can claim that our emotions are in a continuous state of harmony or that we understand why we feel as we do. The key is the everyday mind. I have talked about this concept in the preceding chapters but it is important to remember that the everyday mind is the survival mechanism we develop to get through the ups and downs of daily life in this incarnation as human beings. It is built up of behavior, habits, and strategies we have learned over the years in response to people, events, and situations. It is clever, informed, and cunning, but the everyday mind knows very little about itself. In other words, it is not bad but it is ignorant; although it has enabled us to survive, it does not always act in our best interests.

Behind the everyday mind lies our inner wisdom. This is

the foundation of all living creatures. It is pure consciousness. Our emotions arise from our everyday minds. Emotions are submerged frequencies of energy that undulate in reaction to the way we respond to the world around us and force their way into our waking consciousness. Take a very simple example: It's a sunny day, people smile and say hello, and you feel happy. Emotions are also capable of more sophisticated reactions to others that are sometimes called telepathy. We can, for instance, sometimes sense other people's unhappiness, even if they are far away and we can't see or hear them. Absent healing is another example. Such apparently paranormal experiences are made possible by the effect of these waves of energy.

Bridging the chasm between the everyday mind and the inner wisdom or consciousness is the linchpin of good health, according to Tibetan medical wisdom. Your everyday mind is the catalyst and cause of illness, as it creates behavior that binds you to thoughts and actions that in turn cause you pain and illness.

Knowing how to interpret your emotional energy as an indicator of the state of your consciousness is a great asset. Most of the time our minds and bodies are trying, in vain, to communicate with each other. This blocked communication often creates conflict and disharmony that come out in the shape of anxiety, moodiness, depression, bad temper, shyness, fear, and a range of other negative emotions. This then leads to illness of all kinds. You can see the results of frustrated mind-body communication in such common symptons as tension headaches, work-related neck and back ache, stomach problems, colds, and skin conditions. Most Western scientists now agree that emotions play a major part in many serious illnesses, including cancer and heart disease.

If we can cultivate deeper connections between the body and the mind, we calm the cycles of confusion and then have a greater chance of health.

Tibetan emotional healing is a process that uses a combination of your everyday mind and your inner wisdom to understand how you become ill and also how you can recover and stay well. This requires courage, faith in yourself and the awareness that you are the originator of your states of health and in charge of your healing process.

If you can see deeply enough within your personality, you will start to understand how any condition, emotional or physical, is caused and how it affects you. This knowledge may not heal you in an obvious way, such as improving physical symptoms, but understanding the nature of any condition leads to opportunities to create well-being.

Emotional healing enables a person who feels under pressure to become clear-minded and relaxed, in order to deal with the requirements of everyday living. It can also be used to clear the mind so that a person can have direct experience of his or her inner perfection and, further, to gain insight into intellectual or worldly concerns.

The healing is based on understanding seven simple principles, applying these to the key human experiences, and then using specific meditations to stimulate the healing process.

The Seven Principles

1. Your physical body is still your mind: It is simply the material form of the emotional energy of your mind. Pain, illness, and well-being are the products of your everyday mind. Your inner, unstained true mind holds all understanding to your health and suffering.

2. Reality is not what it seems: Your everyday mind gets its information about the physical world through your senses, but you can't always trust this version. Your senses are taking in information that in seconds

becomes the past. So, your mind is creating a reality that is seemingly in the moment but is really in the past. Understanding this fundamental fact of life enables you to become aware of how situations are created and develop so that you can intuitively sense the way in which one situation gives rise to another.

3. All of our experiences, past and present, influence the nature and quality of emotional and physical health. They are markers in the way our life energy develops and grows. By understanding and transforming the quality of your life experiences, you reduce the possibility of illness. Left unhealed and misunderstood, they may lead to illness and also affect how well you recover. The way you react to feeling ill is also based on all your experiences and how you responded to illness in the past.

4. Illness or any major crisis in your life is mostly a process of the past catching up with you. This does not include natural events such as earthquakes, floods, or accidents, but in many cases, the effects of our past thoughts, actions, and interactions with other people influence how and why we become ill. If we can identify the sources of illness or any major crisis, we can start to extinguish the negative forces of the past and transform them into positive experiences.

5. Your physical body is an expression of consciousness and of all time and space in miniature, a microcosm of the macrocosm. You can help your body develop into a higher state of physical intelligence, which enables it to heal itself. This state of body directly and simply expresses the energies of the mind into the world, thereby bringing peace and harmony. This experience unites us with the divine grace of the uni-

verse and the god or gods of our understanding, teaching us to honor the lives we have entered and guiding us through difficulties.

In this state, you have a direct understanding of the space between moments and you are able to know reality directly and intimately. Just as your mind can experience this enlightenment, so your body can become the physical expression of it. There is no one way in which enlightenment presents itself, because each person's body and mind are unique. Your experience would be different from mine and the next person's, but we would all share common qualities.

6. You can heal your mind and body and achieve dynamic well-being by using the pure state of your inner mind. To do this it is necessary to discipline your everyday mind, which will always try to dominate any interchange that involves the conscious connection between it and your body.

You can start to discipline your everyday mind by observing the way you react to problems:

- Does your body tense up?

- Does your mind go blank or wish the problem would just go away?

- Do you worry or panic?

- Do you feel overwhelmed by the force of the problem?

If you go through these or similar reactions of your body, mind, or spirit, start directing comfort and love to each one. Through this gentle self-help, you will start to understand your reactions and feel more ordered mentally. You will also start to direct the interchange between your body and your mind.

As your everyday mind ceases to try to control your life, you will experience the unfolding of the purity and innocence that is within everyone.

7. Healing in its outer physical form is a subjective experience; the body may take longer than the mind to understand and manifest healing.

The Cyclical Nature of Body and Mind

Tibetan medicine is acutely aware of the importance of the cyclical nature of emotional pain and how this cycle can be used to treat those suffering emotional disturbances and physical illness. All things in the body and mind work on monthly cycles influenced by the moon and the sun. Most are active at certain hours of the day and night, and are also associated with the phases of the moon. So, certain conditions of the mind or body will respond to treatment at certain times of the night and day, in accordance with the individual's inner timing system.

We can tune in to these cycles by doing a modern version of a traditional Tibetan practice. You will first need to get a calendar that shows you the four stages of the moon. These can often be found in New Age shops; alternatively, some newspapers and magazines have astronomy or astrology columns that detail the lunar phases.

The ancient Tibetans believed that on the days of the new and the full moon, lunar energy gathers at the back of your head where it meets your neck. So on these days, take some quiet time and start to tune in to your body. Late evening or early morning is the best time, although any time will do. Focus your mind on that area at the base of your skull and feel the energies of the moon flowing with the tides of your heart, circulation, and breathing.

This is a safe and simple meditation that puts you directly in touch with the cyclical energies of your body and mind. This preparation will help you do all the other meditations in this book.

Painful Human Experiences

According to the Tibetan belief, there are ten main categories of painful human experience. All human beings in all cultures and societies will go through these kinds of emotional pain in some way and at some time in their lives.

1. Anxiety about financial security

2. Anxiety and stress related to physical safety, leading to loss of ability to trust

3. Excessive talking and fear of being alone, stemming from exhaustion

4. Problems of addiction, unskillful behavior of any kind

5. Emotional disturbance caused by environmental influences

6. Problems with family and friends

7. Recurrent bad dreams or nightmares, confusion about time

8. Emotional pain concerned with violence

9. Emotional pain resulting from physical pain

10. Fear of death and dying

By exploring these ten key experiences, we can loosen the mind-made restrictions that encourage us to suffer and to be ill.

Tibetan medicine believes that negative or oppressive energies contain within them the essence of positive and liberating experiences. Simply, what makes you sick or fearful also has the potential to make you well and courageous. You need to turn the negative experience into a positive outcome, and you can do this with the aid of the meditation exercises explained in the following pages.

Bearing in mind the seven principles detailed earlier in this chapter, allow yourself to explore which of the areas of emotional pain affect you and then practice the relevant meditation. Always make yourself as comfortable as you can when you do these exercises. Have a blanket nearby in case you get cold, and plenty of drinking water because you are likely to get thirsty.

Of course, it may be that none of the categories applies to you now, but at some time they will. They may also be of use to other people in your life.

1. Anxiety About Financial Security

This is a universal fear, regardless of culture, time, or place. According to Tibetan spirituality, it is one of the major causes of emotional disturbance and a strong contributor to poor health. Even people who have great wealth worry in this way, which causes their inner natures to be starved of feelings of abundance, nourishment, and safety. This is emotional poverty, a kind of spiritual virus that, like all forms of emotional disturbance, can be transmitted to other people.

Having this anxiety reduces vital life energy and makes you feel unhappy and isolated. And the more you worry about this, the more the worry acts as an obstacle to stop you from changing your situation.

The reason why people worry so much about this aspect of living is, perhaps, that they identify themselves with their belongings. Then they imagine themselves without their possessions, and, more important, they identify themselves with being out in the cold and starving to death. Incredible inner dramas are acted as people create fears that suffuse them with the belief that they deserve no better.

At this very moment, there are millions of people in the world in desperate physical poverty and millions in extreme emotional poverty. Those in physical need can be helped, but those in emotional need will find it harder to change.

Have you ever been weighed down in this way? Have you worried when the money would come? Whether you would have enough to pay the rent, the bills? It is a common experience.

For those of us who are fortunate enough to have our bellies full every day, the inner poverty seems to grow the more we become seduced by our own comfort. Underneath most people's everyday minds lies a fear of losing what we have—job, house, life-style—and never regaining it. Then we become frightened.

This fear comes from a lack of inner connection to our own inner wisdom and our relationship with the natural world.

The material world will give you what you ask of it. Sometimes you will have to struggle to get what you have asked for. At other times, things will come easily. Like the phases of an illness, one day you feel good, the next sick again. But there is a cure for this anxiety.

MEDITATION

The ancient Tibetans believed that you gain something only by giving up something else. But if you feel you have nothing, what do you give up? You give up the nothing you have.

Think about it. In your mind you are anxious about losing everything and having nothing. This means that in your thoughts you possess nothing, with a lot of emotional energy. So, here is how you give it up:

Make yourself warm and sit in a comfortable position. Be quiet and breathe normally.

Let yourself feel the fears you have about your material world. As you feel each one, use your own words to give it up. Let it go. Give them all up to the world around you. Send them away as gently as you can.

Then, tell them to come back to you only when they have become powerful, healing, abundance-making thoughts. In giving them up and demanding that they change, you send strong inner messages to yourself to start generating a new reality.

This meditation is a simple version of what is called a "ransom ritual" in Tibetan culture. You are exchanging negative energy for positive.

Rest in this state of mind, breathe it into you, and think of it as water washing over you. Rest again. As you inhale and exhale, think of each breath as a gentle but penetrating flame burning away all the emotional garbage inside you. Rest. Receive the returning positive energies.

Conditions helped by this meditation:

- Emotional: panic attacks, obsessive greed, jealousy, anger, depression, physical pain with no cause, hysteria, loneliness, lethargy.

- Physical: breathing difficulties, muscle spasms in the chest, stress-related disorders, respiratory and pulmonary problems, bleeding gums that don't respond to treatment, skin problems, digestive disorders.

Jacob was an international criminal. He consulted me for a physical condition and ended up talking about his fear of poverty. He had grown up in the slums of a South American country, living on the streets and scraping together anything

he could to survive. Crime was his way out. He made a
great deal of money and saw himself as a hero of the slums.
But the money did not conquer his ingrained fear of poverty.
He made more and more but still the fear was there. It took
Jacob over two years of practicing this meditation to over-
come his profound insecurity. He put himself to the test by
giving up crime and devoting the money he had made to
help street children. Then he turned himself in to the police.
Jacob has left prison now and works in slums helping the
children there.

2. Anxiety and Stress Related to Physical Safety, Leading to Loss of Ability to Trust

For many people the world is an unsafe place. They may live in war zones, experience horrific violations, or see what they value destroyed. Then, they forget the natural ability to trust. Regardless of what causes the fear, this is an experience that damages personal integrity and well-being and causes extremely poor health and unhappiness.

If you have felt physically unsafe—even for a moment—you know how it feels not to be able to trust people and to think that the world is a bad place. Like the fear of not having enough money, it causes people to hide away their potential and destroys creativity.

The world can overpower such vulnerable people. Having to deal with this constant anxiety can make them self-obsessed and prevent them from communicating openly with others. Most of us have experienced it to some degree: You can see it in the way you guard yourself against other people.

Healing this anxiety empowers you and gives you control over your world.

MEDITATION

Sit in an easy way with no strain on your body, or lie on your back. As you breathe, imagine the breath is flowing in and out through your navel.

Think of the breath flowing to every part of you and your body becoming warmer and more energetic. Then, focus on your physical heart. Imagine that in it lies an image of yourself where you are perfectly safe and free from all harm. Try to allow yourself to blend completely with this image.

Now use your mind to direct this image out into the everyday world around you. Allow it to radiate like sunlight into every corner of your life. Rest, and let yourself receive the good feelings that come to you from doing this.

Conditions helped by this meditation:

- Emotional: speech impediments, communication problems, phobias of any kind, including fear of open or closed spaces, water, or being under ground.

- Physical: spinal and joint-mobility problems, bladder infections, skin problems, discharge from the eyes.

Simon was a bodyguard, intelligent, tough, and very dangerous. He routinely defended his clients from terrorists, assassins, and snipers. His body was covered in scars and so was his mind. Deep inside, he felt scared—of physical violence and of how other people judged him. He trusted no one. His relationships foundered because he could not trust his girlfriends to trust him. Then a friend of his was seriously hurt on a job and Simon blamed himself. He fell to pieces. As he started to unravel his life with the help of this meditation, he discovered that all his martial and psychological skills were defenses to protect him from a frightening world.

*Slowly he let go of his fears and found that he no longer
wanted to work as a bodyguard. The former tough guy found
he had a burning passion for flowers and became a florist.*

3. Excessive Talking and Fear of Being Alone, Stemming from Exhaustion

Why do so many people talk too much? Because they are so
incredibly fatigued in mind and body that they do not know
how to be in their own company if they stop talking and rest in
silence.

They chat to cover up their exhaustion. But because they
do not know how to stop being tired, or are afraid of admitting
how tired they are, they feel themselves compressed into a
small inner space. They also fear spending time on their own
and are unable to acknowledge their inner natures as wonderful beings.

Do you talk too much or get into cycles when your chatter
goes into overdrive? Would you rather be with other people at
all costs than spend time knowing who you are? Discovering
your true self does not have to be an intense spiritual activity; it
can be as simple as this meditation exercise. By integrating this
into your daily life, you can experience the value of both speech
and silence.

MEDITATION

Make yourself comfortable, sitting on a chair with your hands
on your lap. Close your eyes and breathe normally. Start to listen to all the sounds around you. Listen to them whether they
are pleasant or not. Listen without prejudice. Treat them as
your friends.

Each and every sound has something to offer you. Listen.
Soon all the different sounds will merge together.

When this happens, breathe in and out slowly, imagining

that the sounds are flowing into you, moving through your body, into your tongue and your brain, and then out into the world around you. Rest in the silence that comes behind the sounds.

Conditions helped by this meditation:

- Emotional: fearfulness, lack of self-esteem, feeling that the world is grinding you down, feeling constantly overwhelmed.

- Physical: chronic illness of any kind, inner-ear problems, tinnitus, sinus problems, influenza, skin problems, structural problems of the lumbar spine, shoulder pain.

Lara was a motormouth. Nothing could stop her talking, and while some of what she said was meaningful, most of it was rubbish. She told me that she talked all the time because she was afraid of what was inside her. Some people talk to cover up what they perceive as a vacuum, but Lara felt there was something inside, some power, and it so scared her that she covered it up by making noise. As she did the meditation exercise above, she began to feel connected to other people and to herself. She discovered that she was in fact very perceptive and had strong intuitive powers. Within a year she had changed into a person who felt she had to speak only when she had something to say. She now works as a lawyer and uses the meditation to help clients heal their exhausted minds.

4. Problems of Addiction, Unskillful Behavior of Any Kind

Addiction and unskillful behavior of any kind are the emotional fallout from a spiritual crisis. Chemical and psychological addicting are the same, according to Tibetan medical teachings. Unskillful behavior is any thought or action that causes you or someone else pain of any type. Addiction is its own pain and comes about because the person's soul is in a state of shock and disrepair. The emotional structures that enabled the individual to live in the normal world have fallen apart because a great sense of separation and loss has been experienced. This may happen because of repeated unhappiness of any type that creates damage within the person so that he feels unable to make sense of himself, the reality he inhabits, or the rest of the world.

Many addicts are highly developed spiritually but never had the chance to fully develop their inner wisdom. It's as though their minds and bodies cannot handle their inner spiritual awareness, and they quite simply crack open. And they feel that, like Humpty-Dumpty, they can never be put together again.

Addicts use their addictions to avoid confronting their true feelings. This results in a kind of automatic response being set up where they use the same emotional patterns in all circumstances. An alcoholic, for example, would use the pain of dealing with everyday life as a reason for drinking—anything from an argument with a loved one to problems at work. There would always be a justification. The alcohol would appear to hide the pain, but in fact it would just transform it into emotional fuel to drive the alcoholic through another day.

Meditation that enables the pain to heal is a crucial part of a larger recovery process. This exercise empowers the desire to heal the emotional pain coming from addiction and creates a sense of well-being. It helps people to come to terms with the fact that they have an addictive illness; it is also beneficial for those suffering a terminal illness.

MEDITATION

Lie on your back, stretch out, and breathe normally. Focus on your physical heart and listen to your heartbeat.

Now, focus on your addiction. See your addiction pulsing through you in time with the beat of your heart. Through the beat feel the outer limits of your physical body. See how your addiction and your body react to each other. Breathe this in and out.

Direct as much love as you can to the reaction between your body and the addiction. Remember that although your addiction is a spiritual crisis, it is played out within your body through your emotional energy. Now, be as still as you can.

Feel the love you created. Receive as best you can the feelings that you experience as a result of this exercise.

Conditions helped by this meditation:

- Emotional: total despair, desire for suicide or violent behavior to others, sudden fits of crying or rage, obsession with negative experiences.

- Physical: eases the physical pain of nerve damage or terminal illness; encourages the body to rest and allows a better chance for the body's healing systems to work; may help circulatory, elimination, and digestive functions; stops or reduces stress headaches.

Darryl was an addict of epic proportions. He was unable to resist alcohol, drugs, sex, shopping, and his own ego. He tried to give up many times and failed. Partly because he was also addicted to being an addict, it became his raison d'être. He told me that he really wanted to give up but just didn't know how. He felt powerless. Although, like all addicts, he behaved as if he cared nothing for others, in fact he was extraordinarily perceptive about them. And what he felt was so painful that he fell back into his addictions. As he used the meditation, he noticed that he was less affected by other people and the world around him. He felt strong enough to go to his therapist regularly and attend a support group, both of which helped him to deal with the causes of his addiction. He is happier today and works as a therapist.

5. Emotional Disturbance Caused by Environmental Influences

Environmental influences can cause damage in several ways. Being confined either by land or by buildings can lead to emotional disturbance. Physical illness can result from ingesting toxins in the earth, water, plants, gases, or other naturally occurring substances. Additionally, the mind and emotions may become disturbed by the influences of weather, light, wind, and seasonal variations. The Tibetans believe that many people can be adversely influenced in this manner, and that their personalities then take on the prevailing emotional influences created by other people around them.

Cities are regarded as potential sources of emotional pollution because they hold huge amounts of thoughts and energies that can cause people to become confused and to experience increased stress and negative behavior. The way buildings are planned also affects emotional health. Because cities are normally a jumble of conflicting architectural styles, they can block energetic flow.

Certain alignments of natural landscapes can also affect some people's emotional health. Living close to rivers or oceans, for example, can influence stability.

Sometimes a move may be the only solution, but the meditation exercise below can help you to become more balanced and be less influenced by the surrounding environment.

MEDITATION

Make sure you are warm, then lie down on your back. Breathe in and out slowly, as deeply as you can but in your normal manner. Slowly think about how your environment influences you. As you do this, sing the sound *Ahh* over and over again at a deep pitch. Do this quietly at first, then progressively louder.

Imagine that the sound is starting to flow out to every part of your environment, transforming all the negativity and in its place creating a positive healing force that flows back into you so that the environment can no longer influence you. As the positive force flows back to you, imagine that your body and mind start to fill with clear, sparkling energy. Rest, then send this energy back out to the surrounding environment.

Think of everything around you—people, land, and buildings—becoming blessed with overwhelming joy and love. Rest, then send this energy back into the surrounding environment. Once again, think of everything around you—people, land, and buildings—becoming blessed with overwhelming joy and love. Receive this, too, and bless yourself.

Then send this blessing out into the environment and let it go: Do not expect to have it back. Be selfless.

Conditions helped by this meditation:

- Emotional: feeling overwhelmed by your environment in a negative, brooding way; feeling that you have no energy left to do anything—even thinking is too much; feeling sad without knowing why; feeling that you cannot trust, love, or laugh anymore.

- Physical: stomach pains, joint pains, circulatory problems, infectious and viral illnesses, symptons of food poisoning, illnesses caused by any type of parasite, effects of bites by poisonous animals, following orthodox medical treatment.

Geoff lived in the center of one of the world's biggest cities. His senses were dominated by noise, pollution, steel, and glass. The only time he experienced silence and peace was in his twenty-fourth-floor apartment. Although he was a successful writer, counselor, and self-help trainer, he felt exhausted by the city and its noise and tensions. Just walking among the crowds jarred his nerves and drained his energy. He started to feel burned out and withdrawn. At first he thought he was having a breakdown, then he understood that he was suffering from emotional and environmental pollution. The energies of other people and his environment were causing him to lose little pieces of himself. The force of the city and its repressed emotional energies were making him into someone else.

He started to practice the meditation above and within a few months he became more balanced and less influenced by his environment. He also understood that in his desire to help others and be successful in his career, he had not developed sufficient inner resources to deal with all the demands that others placed on him, and that he placed on himself. He realized that his physical environment mirrored the way he felt. His apartment lay in the shadow of a much taller building—just as he felt shadowed.

Geoff had always believed that he could follow his career only in the city, but he decided to move to the nearby countryside. He found that he started to respond to people differently and his clients treated him with new respect. Not only did he feel completely restored, but, to his amazement, he was even more successful.

6. Problems with Family and Friends

Virtually all of us have suffered emotional pain caused by friends and family. There are three types of emotional pain that are common, whatever the culture or circumstance:

- Recurrent emotional pain caused by betrayal of trust

- Emotional pain caused by loneliness and abandonment

- Emotional pain caused by dominating personalities

The following meditation will help to heal the wounds.

MEDITATION

Lie on your back and focus on your body. Feel your physical body and relax into it. Feel its shape, contours, and weight. Feel how heavy you can be. Feel how long your body is, and how strong.

Sense the clear, vibrant energy flowing into your body. Now remember every important person in your life and direct this energy to each of them. It purifies them and removes their pain, fear, and insecurity. It makes them happy.

Now feel all your inner pain starting to melt away as a result of your good thoughts. Slowly you feel more capable and more aware of what is important in your life. Direct these good thoughts out into the world.

Conditions helped by this meditation:

- Emotional: feelings of not being paid enough attention, of abandonment, of being unable to show affection; overwhelming fears of childbirth, sexual intimacy, being alone, being touched.

- Physical: extreme skin conditions including boils, cuts, and wounds, preparing for and recovering from major surgery; terminal illness.

Shara was afraid of everything. Since childhood she had lived with all sorts of emotional pain. Her family had effectively abandoned her—they were, in her words, more inter-

ested in TV than in her—and she was left to wander the
streets. Her conviction that she was stupid and the belief
that no one cared for her dominated her life. She became
involved with prostitution, drugs, and crime. Curiously, it
was a television program that started her journey out of her
personal hell. The show described the lives of people in her
situation and motivated her to get the education she had
never had. During this process Shara also learned about
herself and realized that, despite the strides she had made,
she was still a mess inside. A friend introduced her to me and
she started the meditation exercise. As she practiced it, she
gained great insight into her situation. Her emotional
strength grew and her mind became more alive. She con-
sulted a psychotherapist regularly, and this led to her feeling
that she could start the process of forgiving her family.
Eventually Shara persuaded her parents and her siblings to
practice the meditation with her. The chasm between them
began to close.

7. Recurrent Bad Dreams or Nightmares, Confusion About Time

This type of emotional pain relates to when we are confused,
shocked, perplexed, or blocked by recurrent dreams whose
meanings seem to escape us. It also relates to being frightened
by nightmares or to the sense of being in a dreamlike state
when we are awake, with never enough time to do anything.

The Tibetans believe that dreams hold important spiritual
meanings for us and that we dream in order to maintain sanity
and mental clarity. It is the everyday mind's way of clearing out
emotional garbage, gaining self-knowledge, and learning to
know the true inner mind.

According to Tibetan tradition, our dreams can be culti-
vated so that we can enter into the dream state and discover

the sources of our illusions, delusions, inspirations, and insights. Dreaming is essential in regulating the underlying cycles of health, and this meditation can help to solve problems associated with it.

MEDITATION

Go to bed one hour before you normally do. As you relax, think of a milky-white glowing light beginning to flood through your mind and all your thoughts. All you think and feel and see within is this milky whiteness. Time has no place: You understand that it is artificial.

Focus on a recurring dream or nightmare. As you start to feel or see it, let it start to dissolve into the milky whiteness. Allow a great feeling of peace to flow through you. Time washes away like paint in water.

Out of the whiteness comes the true meaning or indication of your dream or nightmare. You are freed of time. Let it go.

Then, allow yourself to fall asleep. You will start to discover a new way of dreaming.

Conditions helped by this meditation:

- Emotional: feeling emotionally stuck, unable to make decisions or speak clearly; feeling controlled by time and all its associated experiences and problems.

- Physical: difficulty in waking, poor vision and sense of smell, hair loss, weight problems, sore throats, rheumatic conditions, bladder and liver problems, minor glandular problems, wasting of muscles; it can also help the well-being of patients with osteoarthritis, metastatic tumors, lymphoma (cancers of the lymph system), and Paget's disease (a chronic bone-wasting condition).

Every night, John, a soldier who had seen active duty in war zones, would dream of a young child who was crying silently. All around there were scenes of war and pestilence, famine and disease. The child would start to radiate light and fly on angelic wings over the dead and dying, sprinkling water over them in a blessing.

John would wake in tears and in physical pain. All he could think about was the dream. Paradoxically, he felt as if his everyday life were a dream. When he started to do the meditation he became more open and aware of conflicts between his inner self and his job. As he spoke to me about it, he realized that his inner spirit was calling him to face the anguish and horror of what he had witnessed during his active service. He felt a rising conflict between his spiritual needs and his life in the armed forces. Then, as he was going through old photographs one day, he saw the face of the child in his dream. It was him as a young child.

Suddenly John knew what he had to do. Despite scorn from some of his colleagues, he became a chaplain, tending to the spiritual needs of people in the armed forces. He became a spiritually empowered person who, through his own experience, was able to bring spiritual insight into the lives of those who wanted it.

8. Emotional Pain Concerned with Violence

Violence is a state of active confusion that seeks to control forces beyond it. I am talking here about violent feelings in your mind, about violent action that you take against others or is taken against you.

Violence is based not on anger but on greed. Greed wants to control, separate, and divide. Violence destroys what is around it and also destroys its originator. But violence and greed are within all of us, an essential activating energy that can be transformed. Greed seeks to be listened to before it will transform itself into positive energy; violence seeks only to be acknowledged by all those involved in the violent act so that it may transmute into love and wisdom.

Emotional pain caused by violence is a form of energetic injury, a spiritual bruising that can be healed by meditation.

MEDITATION

Lie on your back and relax. Focus your mind on your belly. Feel yourself becoming physically stronger. Rest in this sensation and allow it to flow all over your body.

Focus on the emotional pain caused by violence. Direct the physical sensations of strength into your pain and let it start to dissolve. In its place see a deep copper-red light flow all over your body and flood into your mind. This light cascades into your physical heart, which pumps it, through your veins, throughout your body, bones, and brain.

Rest in this state for as long as you are able.

Conditions helped by this meditation:

- Emotional: releasing the experience of reliving a physical trauma; sudden negative thoughts that come out of nowhere.

- Physical: muscle damage and general mobility problems of the upper body.

Dorothy, a doctor, came to see me because she had experienced violence firsthand and felt she could not continue living. She had worked with child prostitutes, pimps, drug dealers, and other dangerous people in a poverty-stricken area of a large city.

She was caught up in a riot that flared when the police raided someone's house. Caught in the crossfire, she was shot in the chest and legs. As she tried to get up, she was stabbed repeatedly and had her jaw and arm broken. A friend who lived in the slum came to her rescue, persuading the police to take her to a hospital.

Dorothy was much respected and both sides apologized after they realized who she was, but the harm had been done. Her body had taken on the injury and the pain. She gave up her work in the city and practiced in a quieter area. But the violence continued inside her.

She was so traumatized that she cut herself off from her husband and children. She was afraid to go out by herself and wanted to stop being a doctor. She couldn't understand why it had all happened to her. She felt angry, powerless, and violated.

Dorothy learned the meditation and bit by bit her shock began to heal. It also helped the constant pain from her injuries. An excellent psychotherapist, who encouraged her to continue the meditation, also helped, and she was eventually able to forgive those who had hurt her. The last I heard of her, she was still practicing medicine and had felt secure enough to visit the slum where the violence had occurred.

9. Emotional Pain Resulting from Physical Pain

Extreme or constant physical pain can cause our emotions to close down, which restricts the process of healing or recovery. The emotional pain is experienced as stress, worry, anxiety, or other forms of emotional restriction. It serves only to prolong physical pain, thus creating a vicious cycle. The emotional pain becomes harder and harder to deal with because it is just the tip of whatever physical pain you are experiencing.

MEDITATION

Sit as comfortably as you can. Listen to your breathing and follow your breath as it flows in and out; focus on the short natural pause between the inhalation and exhalation.

As you breathe in, feel huge amounts of powerful positive energy flowing into every part of you, softening your pain and reducing its intensity. As you breathe out, let your pain flow out, leaving your body soft and warm.

With every breath, feel your pain reduce and your body increase in mobility and warmth. Warmth flows everywhere in your mind and body. Gently it turns into a radiant sky blue, and your body and mind are flooded with this sparkling sky-blue light. Your physical pain is released.

Now rest, and give goodness to all living creatures so that they too can reduce their pain.

Conditions helped by this meditation:

- Emotional: seeing beyond the experience of pain to understand its nature, why you have it, and that you can control or manage it; fear caused by pain.

- Physical: extreme oversensitivity due to nerve damage; regulates uneven breathing, thus helping pain levels; digestion and excretion.

Sam had been in constant pain all his life because of nerve damage from a childhood car crash. Depression and mood swings were his everyday state. For a time, he was addicted to painkillers. As his physical pain fueled his emotional pain, his suffering became more intense. Normal relationships with other people were difficult because the pain made his body twitch, which made him feel like a freak. His emotions became frozen and he started to hate the world and to with-

draw from people. A friend explained this meditation to him and also encouraged him to come and see me. As Sam learned the meditation, he started to let go of the emotions that the pain had trapped in his body and mind through the years. Feelings came back to his mind, and, as they did so, the physical pain lessened. Today, the pain has greatly improved with the effect of the meditation. He still uses it regularly to help his body and mind move toward knowing his inner wisdom.

10. Fear of Death and Dying

According to Tibetan teachings, death does not happen in the way we in the West think it does. Our bodies cease, but our inner natures continue. Life after life, the qualities of our inner natures adapt to the differing experiences of each life, in much the same way as our minds adapt to each circumstance in this life.

The Tibetans teach that fears surrounding death and dying stem from fears about what we may discover about ourselves as we go through the death experience.

Understanding the brevity of physical life helps you to respect your mind, your body, and other people. But a lot of people flash from one life to another without realizing that they go through the process of dying. As in life, they rush through, without cherishing or knowing it. The fear of death and dying comes because you are in some way aware of the process within you, but you have not accepted it.

When fears about death get out of hand, it is because the person concerned has had some insight into his or her spiritual nature, which heightens the awareness of impermanence. Such people are often psychic, empathic, or highly intuitive, and also acutely aware of other people's suffering. But because their minds are not trained to deal with this awareness, they can become confused and unable to make sense of their own lives.

This meditation will help to still the conflict.

MEDITATION

This exercise shows you the life-giving energy behind the nature of death. It also slightly mimics what people experience as they die.

Be as still as you can. Let your breathing slow down. Imagine that all your senses and thoughts can pick up and see everything around you. You may feel a little overwhelmed. Do not worry. Be at peace.

You can sense a clear, sparkling light flowing around you. Imagine that you want to speak to those who care for you, but they can't hear your voice. You feel as if you're in a fast-moving river, being jostled about. You get near the edge of a waterfall and fear you may fall over, but you don't. You stay safely on the edge, suspended in space.

You start to become aware of just how many people are being born and dying at this very moment. All you sense is joy and happiness. There is no fear.

Relax into this feeling and receive its energy. You see a clear light come toward you. Enter into it without doubt and stay there for as long as you can.

When you leave the light, rest and give thanks for all parts of nature and life. Send love and goodness to all life.

Conditions helped by this meditation:

- Emotional: the need always to be in control, arrogance; effects of gossip on both the gossiper and the person talked about; inability to share emotions, money, or insight; doubts about loving and love; fears of finding out who you are and of living the life that is true for you, of taking responsibility for your life, of growing up; fear that at death there is nothing else.

- Physical: problems of the neck and spinal structure of
  the neck, problems of the jaw and upper and lower
  palate; thrombosis, angina, cardiac conditions, her-
  nias, vomiting, problems following exposure to severe
  elements; helpful after transplants and in easing
  shock or injury to the head.

*Dan was a Catholic priest who also worked as a psycho-
therapist. When I met him, he was going through a crisis
of faith because he had discovered he was afraid of death
and dying. He tried to deal with his fear by exerting
a fierce control over his life. The repercussions had
started to contaminate his emotions and his relationships
and to affect his body—his jaw became rigid and very
sore and his back tensed up and caused him pain. As the
fear got worse, Dan lost all his connection with living:
Life was something that happened to other people. A
close friend told Dan that he had become callous and
uncaring toward him and others. This shocked him profoundly.*

   *His whole life was meant to be dedicated to caring for
others and serving his God—the God who had con-
quered death. When we met, Dan felt he was powerless
to do anything—carry out his work, connect with the
divine, even walk or listen to music. He was isolated
and lonely.*

   *Practicing this meditation slowly reconnected him to life,
and he began to understand that life includes death. He
began to feel the stirrings of his faith being reborn, and he
started to study death and dying as part of his work. This
enabled him to become a whole person, equipped to help
others to heal their own fears. He uses the meditation as a
form of prayer to help him communicate with his God, his
source of eternal life.*

Dan discovered that, for him, coming to terms with death was the doorway to the meaning of life.

Reflect on this chapter in quiet. Learn how your inner self is responding to the exercises. You will find they improve your sense of harmony and well-being.

You can use these meditations for other people, but be absolutely sure that they want to receive such energies. If possible, ask them directly.

To do the exercises for someone else, think of the person and then do the meditation.

These are powerful healing exercises, so use them with discernment. Every good thought misdirected has an effect somewhere in the world that may be undesirable.

CHAPTER SIX

The Three Humors

The concept of the three humors is at the heart of the operating system of Tibetan medicine. Physicians categorize people into three humoral types: Wind (*rlung*), Bile (*mkhris pa*), and Phlegm (*bad kan*). Physicians see the humors as energetic forces with different characteristics, moving through your body and mind and out into the universe.

- Wind is a clear, sparkling, colorless stream of energy that can be quick or slow or completely still, all at the same time.

- Bile is a dark red-brown bubbling energy, like lava, which is dense yet taut and fast-moving.

- Phlegm is a deep, relaxed, blue-green force that is reflective and very slow-moving.

According to Tibetan medicine, the three humors are the basis of all our experiences, from the time of conception to physical death. They govern every aspect of how the body and mind function, create structures, and talk to one another. They are implicit in all our emotional, intellectual, spiritual, and physical dynamics. They are the centers of our minds and form the embodiment of our personalities. They hold the abundance of who we can be. They can reveal the deepest workings of our own consciousness, both as individuals and as members of the human species. We are never separated from them: As we are born, die, and are recycled in the natural world, so are the three humors.

They interact in this way:

- Wind is the motivating force and life energy of the others, but it cannot act harmoniously without them.

- Wind increases the intensity of the Bile humor's influence.

- Wind gives Phlegm movement and adaptability and enhances its supportive functions in the body.

- Bile stimulates the activity of Wind.

- Bile delivers warmth and action to Phlegm.

- Phlegm can relax Bile.

Each and every human endeavor is created, continued, and destroyed by the dynamic flow of the humors. Like three great currents moving through all humankind, these forces are the origins of our cultural and psychological identities. In a state of balance, they sweep us toward higher thought and actions. Out of balance, they drive us into nightmares of negative and catastrophic activity. By learning to know your humoral nature and harmonizing it, you contribute to the harmony of the world.

We are predominantly one humoral type, or a combination of two—the first dominant and the second subdominant. But all three humors are within each of us, and the aim is to achieve balance, so that they work together to create well-being and prevent poor health. Although people are far more complex than this kind of typing may suggest, categorizing them in this way helps Tibetan medicine explain how illness expresses itself in individuals and how they experience well-being.

Illness occurs when our dominant humor (and/or the sub-dominant humor, if we have one) is out of balance. This happens principally through life-style problems, including stress, poor diet, and pollution, which make us susceptible to diseases of different types, from colds to cancer.

Good health is based on balancing the humors. By understanding how they adapt, react, and condition their environment—that is, you—you will become more aware of how you create patterns that reduce well-being and lead to illness, and the reverse. This process can take place on many inner levels, connected to many everyday experiences.

The Origins of the Three Humors

Tibetan Bön legend ascribes the origins of the theory to the first inhabitants of the earth—nonhuman beings who are known as the nineteen brothers and sisters of existence. Medical anthropologists and experts on Tibetan culture believe the theory traveled with traders and migrating peoples into Tibet and the Himalayan region from Central Asia in the ninth century B.C. or even earlier.

The legend carried into Tibet and the Himalayan region, eventually finding its way into the Indian subcontinent to influence Vedic beliefs, and then Hinduism and the Indian medical system known as Ayurveda. The theory then returned to Tibet in the seventh and eighth centuries A.D. with the arrival of Indian Buddhist missionaries.

The three humors are also reflected in the Western theory of the four cardinal humors. Hippocrates, a doctor working on the

Greek island of Cos, in the early fifth century A.D., put forward the theory that the body had four humors, which were the chief fluids of the body: black bile (also known as melancholy or black choler), yellow bile (or choler), blood, and phlegm. This signaled a new approach to medicine as a natural science; baleful deities had formerly been held responsible for illness and disease. It's likely that Hippocrates based his belief on the system of the three humors.

The expression of the three humors is inextricably entwined with the concept of the five elements—Earth, Water, Fire, Wind/Air, and Space—which are in all aspects of consciousness, mental, psychological, physical, and intellectual. The humors are the result of how the elements interact with one another.

The Nature of Illness

Tibetan medicine believes there is a strong psychosomatic relationship in many forms of illness. Why? Because, simply put, your life, my life, all our lives, day in and day out, are psychosomatic experiences. Our psychological nature interacts with the physical world, each affecting the other and creating a continuous new experience that adds up to the quality of our daily lives.

The Tibetans claim that we are born, not brand-new as we believe in the West, but already one year old. Before our first breath, we have been conditioned by our psychosomatic experiences in the womb. There, we experienced the world through our senses of taste and hearing, even sight, so we come into each physical life with certain qualities and habits already influencing our behavior. Some of our basic humoral tendencies are already formed, crucially the way we respond to illness and health.

Tibetan medicine regards illness as an obstruction. Obstructions decrease valuable life energy. If you have a problem that will not go away, or one that continually repeats itself, an obstruction is at the root. What this means is that you have the potential to suffer an illness because the three humors have become damaged and started to throw your body and mind out of balance.

Taking this one step further, Tibetans see problems that affect our minds in the way we think of a physical complaint. The damage that mental problems cause to our well-being is the same as that of a physical wound. To heal this trauma and create well-being, we have to cultivate good attitudes that increase the quantities of physical and mental energies available to us.

The humors are seen as the foundations of anger, lust, and greed (the origins of the eight material activities, as I described in chapter 4). Ignorance of why and how we suffer lulls us into becoming trapped by these three unskillful emotions. This mental ignorance is the basic cause of suffering and of all bodily illnesses, according to Tibetan medicine.

The body is more than blood, muscle, bone, and nerve; it is an extension of the material mind in the everyday world. To become a whole person—mentally, physically, emotionally, and spiritually—you must try to heal your ignorance by caring for the three humors.

As we improve our attitudes—reducing our anger, lust, and greed—our humoral balances improve. In the Tibetan view, the healthy individual is one who can balance the ups and downs of everyday life in such a way that good energy comes in a spontaneous manner.

Well-being and illness are basically the same process, but expressed differently. One can be born from the other. Every day, our minds take in a series of experiences. The way in which our minds and bodies respond to those experiences directs our health. But we have the ability to transform obstructions. If, for example, we encounter problems at every turn but manage to focus on the creation of good energy, the obstructions lose their bite, and we do not become ill.

At the end of this chapter are self-healing exercises to help you to overcome the sort of obstructions we all meet in everyday life.

Identifying and Looking After Your Humoral Type

The theory of the three humors is very complex. If you went to a physician of Tibetan medicine, you would be asked twenty-nine comprehensive questions to diagnose humoral imbalances; depending on your answers, the physician would prescribe remedies. I have simplified this process here to enable you to understand the emotional and psychological aspects of each of the humors and to initiate your own simple self-healing program. In chapter 8, which deals with food and nutrition, you will find more about the medical aspects of the three humors.

The following sections will enable you to learn the general attributes of the three humors, to identify your dominant humor (or combination of dominant and subdominant humors), to investigate any imbalances, and to restore health using the ancient Tibetan wisdom of seasonal healing, which connects you to the cycles of nature through food, environment, and life-style. Don't mix up the seasonal activities, as you would then risk more imbalance: They are quite specific to each humor and season.

You may find that you have a dominant and a subdominant humor; in this case, follow the seasonal activities for your dominant humor. Later, when your dominant humor is balanced, you can begin to work on your subdominant humor.

Understanding the three humors will help you to become more loving, powerful, and generous, to grow a little wiser, and not to take yourself as seriously as society would sometimes have you do. Let your heart be open and your mind clear and discerning so that you may discover the enlightenment that is to be found in the miracle of daily life.

GENERAL GUIDELINES FOR MAINTAINING HUMORAL BALANCE

1. Always follow your inner voice, otherwise known as "intuition," about situations and people.

2. When you are in good health, always eat and drink what you intuitively feel is right for you. Exercise as much as you want, whether that is a little or a lot.

3. Respect other people and other life-forms.

4. Be as good as you can, and do not do anything you believe to be wrong.

5. Follow an occupation that is in accordance with what you truly want and need; personal satisfaction is the best medicine for keeping your humors balanced.

GENERAL FACTORS THAT UNBALANCE THE HUMORS

1. Eating food that disagrees with you in any way; for instance, making you feel heavy or sluggish, bloated, or otherwise uncomfortable.

2. Not giving yourself enough rest and sleep at appropriate times.

3. Not respecting your body and/or mind, whether this means taking them for granted or, more actively, holding them in contempt.

4. Undergoing continual stress that causes changes in your behavior or personality.

5. Acting or behaving in a way that causes you shame or embarrassment or brings hurt to others.

THE NATURE OF WIND HUMOR

The workings of the Wind humor, which is situated in the center of the body, are not always easy to see. Wind is affected by your thought processes, the way the central nervous system communicates with your physical body, and how all the sensory organs perceive and interpret knowledge and relay it back to your brain.

For instance, the way in which your skin—your largest organ—works to protect you against the environment and how it acts as a conduit for sensation are Wind functions.

The Wind humor also influences breathing, heart rate, speech patterns, and general energy levels. It is associated with greed, melancholy, and the type of depression that causes people to lose touch with the world.

If unbalanced, Wind, like Bile (see p. 134), can speed up the process of illness. Stress and negative patterns can cause Wind and Bile to rise, which leads to shortness of breath, shock or trauma, or skin eruptions, or to descend, causing cramps or other problems with the intestines, pancreas, liver, or gall bladder.

Wind shows its effects in the body and mind through dryness and lightness. Wind-dominant people tend to have bony, angular bodies, sometimes crooked-looking. There is thinness about them and a very slight bluish tint to their complexions. Their joints can "crack" or seem a little stiff when moving. They catch colds or chills easily. They love to sing and argue, enjoy dangerous situations and taking risks, and need drama of any type in their lives. They can be extremely sentimental and naive. They like bitter and sour foods and enjoy strong alcoholic drinks.

All children, from birth up to age eleven, are Wind types. After eleven, they separate into the different categories of humor, some staying as Wind types. Wind adults may be very spiritual and apparently happy, yet also depressed at the same time. They teeter on a tightrope. A Wind person whose humor is balanced would, for example, help people without wanting reward or recognition.

Wind people can improve their self-healing abilities by developing mental clarity through meditation or simply stopping and contemplating. This will help them to get in touch with the knowledge that is a powerful resource of energy, both physical and mental, deep inside them. Everything they need is there, just waiting to be discovered.

People who are predominantly Wind with a subdominant Bile are short and often squat, as the two humors together create a powerful interaction and dynamic tension in which the height and thinness of the pure Wind type is overpowered by the emphatic energy of the Bile humor. Wind/Bile types have a tendency to be very fixed on ambition and success. People who have this humoral combination makes natural teachers and negotiators. They are peacemakers and are often seen as examples of human potential.

People who add Phlegm to a dominant Wind humor may be shy but tend to be curious about everything. Adults with this combination tend to be small and very much connected to the natural forces of the planet. There is sometimes a slight golden tint to their hands and feet, while the rest of their skin is light-toned.

Those who have a Wind imbalance typically pester you at parties, talk too much about themselves, and become upset when you leave, or they ask you for money at airports or when you go shopping. Busybodies, gossips, and religious fanatics also come into this category, as do most politicians, because they deal in ideas and talk with very little physical manifestation.

People who work in television and associated media, computer software, and the Internet are good examples of the

Wind humor. They work with unseen energies and communicate with a technology whose essence is invisible to the human eye but which permeates every culture in the world.

Characteristics of Being in Balance

When they are in balance, Wind types are full of energy, highly intuitive, and very willing to help others. They have lithe, strong, supple bodies that they fuel with their preferred diet of fresh fruit and vegetables, plus a little meat and dairy food. They are enchanted by music and dance and are happiest when exploring their spiritual potential.

Wind/Bile personalities share the same characteristics as Wind types when in balance, but are more introverted, with sudden bursts of energy that are highly directed and focused.

Wind/Phlegm types find harmony by immersing themselves in the natural world. Quiet and gentle when in balance, they have a great capacity for understanding the forces of nature and communicating this to others. They understand the natural energy of the planet and are good with plants and animals.

Symptoms of Wind Imbalance

Wind: Sleep problems, dislike of exposed environments, anxiety for no obvious reason, general unhappiness, joint pains, involuntary twitching, wasting of muscles, neurological problems such as Parkinson's disease and dementia, breathing problems, pins-and-needles sensations, sudden bursts of fatigue or energy, and cravings for food, alcohol, drugs, or people.

Wind/Bile: As above, but singly. When out of balance, this combination of humors has a tendency to manifest single symptoms, physical or emotional, that come on suddenly and last only a short time, leaving the Wind/Bile person exhausted.

Wind/Phlegm: As Wind, but in a slow, lingering manner. When out of balance, Wind/Phlegm types become ill very slowly and may have no idea that they have an underlying disease.

How to Heal Wind Imbalances According to the Seasons

Spring: Drink fresh juices at room temperature in the morning. Drink small amounts of dark beer with roasted root vegetables and eat dark meats or oily fish. Spend time looking at the new growth around you and, if you can, work in a garden or on a farm. Massage your feet, legs, hands, fingers, and arms for twenty minutes twice daily; avoid afternoon naps, but do go to bed early.

Summer: Sunbathe for one hour in the afternoon. Take warm baths twice daily for half an hour. Choose peaceful surroundings and supportive friends. Drink freshly made vegetable and fruit juices for breakfast. Avoid eating salads raw—instead, poach vegetables lightly or wilt leaves. Eat roasted root vegetables. Avoid meats, coffee, tea, alcohol, puddings, and sweets.

Autumn: Spend time near running water. Listen to soft music, books read aloud, and the sound of children's laughter (or that of teenagers or adults who are young at heart). Eat little and often and avoid sweet foods and alcohol.

Winter: Play with happy children and healthy dogs. Sit in contemplation near an open fire, but don't get too hot. Burn incense with a calming aroma, such as sandalwood, myrrh, frankincense, jasmine, or any Tibetan incense. Eat warming comfort foods, such as soups and stews, but avoid oversweet or spicy dishes. Evening meals with high-fat foods, accompanied by dark beer, are beneficial. Massage your entire body gently and firmly for twenty minutes when you wake and at bedtime, using sesame seed oil, clarified butter (ghee), or any thick vegetable oil.

THE NATURE OF BILE HUMOR

This is the heating humor, located in the left side of the body, which stimulates digestion and immune functions and controls heart rate, digestion, respiration, and the excretory process, among other bodily functions. Bodily reflexes are also controlled by Bile.

This humor influences anger and laughter. Bile people have a tendency to be cranky, annoyed by small things, and impatient to get things done now—or preferably yesterday. An imbalance can accentuate this attitude.

Bile-dominant people have strong appetites and get hungry and thirsty frequently. There is a very slight red or light yellow tint to their complexions. They are normally acutely intelligent, with a tendency toward mysticism, and may be egotistical and quietly proud.

Bile types with a Phlegm subdominance are normally tall, bony, and nervous, because the two humors are in a love/hate relationship, with Bile constantly overheating the moisture of the Phlegm, while Phlegm is trying to cool down the ardor of the Bile.

In the same way as Wind (see p. 130), Bile can speed up the process of illness. Bile-dominant people are very aware of their individuality. Any type of overactivity, including extreme attitudes and obsessions, increases Bile imbalance. This can be generated by violent energies, such as severe hate, anger, or emotional upset.

Characteristics of Being in Balance

When balanced, Bile types are highly active and are deep and profound thinkers who make natural leaders. They have great endurance and stamina; sports and other challenging activities are a crucial part of their life-style. They are powerfully interested in the opposite sex. They love meats and spicy foods, and tend to eat little and often. They like reading, researching, and debating issues and are capable of inspiring others to be passionate about life.

Bile/Wind types in balance seek to right wrongs and help the downtrodden; they are deeply connected to the ideas of justice, human rights, equality, and freedom for all—this becomes their raison d'être.

When balanced, Bile/Phlegm combinations imbue everyone they meet with a sense of safety and security; they understand the importance of nurturing and of laying down roots and are excellent at creating homes, balanced families, and communities; they are the storytellers and keepers of family histories and heirlooms; they remember the past and pass it on with insight; they are the keepers of community records.

Bile people often use their impressive personal wisdom to benefit others. For example, a Bile person would have no hesitation in saving someone's life without regard for his or her own safety. All emergency services are typically influenced by Bile, also natural events such as earthquakes, tidal waves, lightning and thunderstorms, or the outbreak of war.

The effects of Bile on the mind and body can be pervasive and penetrating and are felt in every part of a person's life.

Symptoms of Bile Imbalance

Bile: Stomach pains, back problems, digestive disorders, constipation, feeling of tiredness just after eating or drinking, recurrent infections or injuries, sexually transmitted diseases, blood disorders, sudden bouts of anger, recurrent bad dreams that cause physical reactions such as waking in a state of alarm, sweating, shouting out loud, and sleepwalking.

Bile/Wind: As above, but this combination experiences short, sharp symptoms that come and go quickly.

Bile/Phlegm: As above, but the symptoms will have a slow onset, become intense, and then linger.

How to Heal Bile Imbalances According to the Seasons

Spring: Aim for light foods, bland and nutritious, such as soups and broths, with weak black tea in the evening, but no coffee. A calm environment is essential, preferably near trees; if this is impossible, pin up photos of mountains and lakes and watch nature programs on TV. Direct but gentle conversations are important. Massage the upper torso and joints twice daily for twenty minutes, on waking and before bed, using an invigorating, strong-smelling oil or balm that does not irritate your skin.

Summer: Again, light foods are important to balance unbalanced Bile. Encourage friendly but honest conversations. Try doing puzzles and crosswords and playing cards or board games—gamble if you wish, but not with money. Do good things for other people and read books that make you feel better spiritually.

Autumn: Do plenty of gentle physical exercise, such as stretching, yoga, or t'ai chi. Take walks in beautiful places and expeditions to museums and galleries. Watch comedy films.

Winter: Massage on waking, before lunch, and before bed for twenty minutes; always massage away from the heart in long, sweeping strokes. A high-protein diet is important, so eat a balanced diet of fish and grains, but no meat of any kind. Choose red and orange fruits and vegetables; apricots are particularly good.

THE NATURE OF PHLEGM HUMOR

Phlegm, which originates in the right side of the chest, is a quiet, deeply placed energetic function that is concerned with holding everything together, physically and mentally. It is best visualized as a slow-moving, clear, sticky glue that binds yet encourages growth. Phlegm influences bones, muscle growth, metabolic functions, and all of the body's major cycles, as well as the nature of how we create memories and what we perceive to be true or false.

Phlegm energy inspires deep thinking and an interest in philosophy, plus a desire for creativity of all sorts, from making money to works of art. In balance, Phlegm types prefer simple, light foods and are happy enabling others to find fulfillment and well-being.

Phlegm types can become imbalanced if they are very shy, overly serious, emotionally locked up, or in denial about their ability to reach a higher sense of happiness or spirituality. As they dress themselves in Phlegmatic overcoats to protect themselves from emotional pain, so they start to erode their bodies' ability to self-heal, and diminish their mental capacities.

Society could not evolve and progress without this humor because it gives us a sense of continuity, history, and cultural awareness. All religious structures are Phlegmatic, as are institutions like banks, stock exchanges, armed forces, and governments.

Charitable organizations, such as the Salvation Army, are Phlegmatic in nature due to their desire to improve people's lives and bring stability. Negative Phlegm influences can be seen in people who allow themselves to be defined by their jobs and in the obstructive red tape of big bureaucracies.

Characteristics of Being in Balance

The Phlegm/Wind combination enables people who uphold tradition and want to create lasting institutions that will help others. They know instinctively how to use material forces for the benefit of society. Phlegm/Wind people tend to be chubby, introverted, brooding, and of average height.

Phlegm/Bile types also respect tradition, but they have no qualms about ripping down outdated traditions and creating waves in general. They are the people who will use their mental energy to create new ways of thinking, employing the written word as their chosen means of communication.

Phlegm-dominant people often feel cold, chilly, or uncomfortable in their bodies, regardless of weather and environment. They have a tendency to put on weight and have pale complexions. They have strong constitutions that act very slowly. Normally they have a long life span. They like sour-tasting foods and drinks and are often smokers.

Phlegm combined with Bile makes a person very sensual, with a leaning to artistic and physical expression. These types are often tall, with lithe bodies, and their skin has a bronze tint to it. They may suffer from a superiority complex and be easily influenced by superficial things.

Symptoms of Phlegm Imbalance

Phlegm: Skin outbreaks and diseases, eye problems, lung disorders, hormonal problems, lack of virility, problems conceiving and in pregnancy, eating disor-

ders, weight problems, bone disorders, depression
that turns to violence, alcohol addiction, mental collapse, burnout from work or other circumstances.

Phlegm/Wind: As above, but this combination experiences one or more symptoms very intensely over a
long time because the Phlegm humor dominates the
healing Wind humor, rather like a brick (Phlegm)
sitting on a feather (Wind) and pinning it down.

Phlegm/Bile: As above, but the symptoms would normally become apparent only at a time of stress.

How to Heal Phlegm Imbalances According to the Seasons

Spring: Eat lots of fish and cooked vegetables, beans
and grains, with a little red meat twice a week. Avoid
alcohol, coffee, and tea. Take a lot of physical exercise, especially swimming, in rivers or the sea, if possible. Spend ten minutes daily in a sauna or steam
room. Massage with a nonirritating, strong-smelling
ointment or balm for forty minutes, three times a
week in the middle of the afternoon. Cooking, bak-
ing, and simply talking to friends around a kitchen
table are healing.

Summer: Aim to live in a warm, dry, gently breezy environment with lovely scenery, beautiful views, and
wide-open spaces. Play romantic music. Stay calm in
the morning and take light activity in the afternoon.
Eat in the same way as for spring. Massage three
times daily for fifteen minutes to one hour before
each meal in a strong, continuous, counterclockwise
movement, using chickpea flour or talc. Go to bed
before 10 P.M. to encourage the body's cycles to
improve the humoral balance.

Autumn: Again, take lots of exercise and eat as in spring and summer, avoiding alcohol, coffee, and tea. Massage yourself with warm oil for one hour on waking, twice a week; always massage down the body from the head to the feet in short, gentle strokes. Take a hot bath for ten minutes in the midafternoon every day.

Winter: Massage as above three times a week on waking. Eat fish and grains, with a little spice in the evenings only, but no meat at all. Avoid salt, which causes further imbalance.

Improving Humoral Balance by Overcoming Obstructions

Once again, Tibetan medicine regards illness as an obstruction that can damage the humors and make you susceptible to illness. However, obstructions of all kinds can be transformed by the use of emotional tools. Below you will find simple descriptions of how to do this in your everyday life.

These tools lead us to examine how we see the everyday material world, with all its pressures and its fragile social structure. The mainstays of our worldview are ourselves, our circumstances, and other people. By understanding how we think about ourselves, we can know how we create the foundations of health and illness. If our attitudes are unbalanced or confused, we run the risk of creating obstructions that prevent us from experiencing mental, physical, and spiritual health.

The starting place is to learn how we relate to other people, what we say, and how other people react to what we say. We also need to assess what the words we choose say about us, when we are speaking in anger, for example, or in the throes of passion, love, or any other emotion.

Attitudes toward our work and how we identify with it are also key to how we set up our relationships with others. Work, in this context, means any activity we undertake with which we identify strongly. For most of us, that means hundreds of daily tasks, big and small.

Stress is a major obstruction these days, but people respond quite differently to the pressure: A sensible person might allow himself to collapse and rest the moment he can, while a more foolish one would fight on and later find himself burned out and ill.

Prejudice, too, can create obstructions. Prejudice of any sort is the opposite of higher thinking: It represses people into states of worthlessness and triviality. Illness, according to Tibetan medicine, is a prejudice that you have created against yourself.

Transforming your view of yourself and your situation in the ways described below can help you to overcome obstructions and create well-being in your life. We all have within us the cures to our problems and illnesses. We are both the medicine and the healer.

TEN INSIGHTS INTO OBSTRUCTIONS

1. Relationships of All Types

People are other people's biggest problem. Think of the number of people you have to deal with every day at home and at work: husbands, wives, children, parents, and other relatives; friends and lovers; colleagues, employees, and bosses; trades people, spiritual advisers, clergy, or other mentors—not to mention the man in the street.

Good communication is the heart of successful relationships. Everyone wonders what makes other people tick, what they're thinking about, and how they can change it. But, so often, we expend huge energy trying to communicate and end up with little to show for it.

The most common type of obstruction lies in communicating clearly and dealing with difficult situations or people. Remember that a difficult person is a difficult situation. This exercise will reduce the problems you experience with people every day.

The ancient Tibetans discovered a simple way to heal poor communication and to establish trust, power, and spiritual abundance. It is this: Sometimes you have to get tough, other times you have to be gentle, and others you need to be neutral. Of course, you have to know what to be at the appropriate time. You can do this by developing a very simple mental skill that will quickly become part of your everyday thinking. It goes like this:

When you are in a meeting or any other situation with other people, listen to them actively. Direct your mental energy into the words that they speak, and you will find that you can see—behind their language—the truth of what they are really saying.

Once you hear the truth behind their words, you know how you should act, whether that is to be tough, neutral, or gentle. This in itself enables you to prevent obstructions from occurring in the first place or to heal existing ones.

Obstacles become obstacles because they are given unskillful energy and so become difficult to move. When you get a response of any kind from an obstacle, it starts to move. Once this happens, you can start to resolve the problem.

2. Employment and Religion

Work, career, or any other activity that is involved in making a living requires the creation of an identity for the worker. That means setting up some kind of power base, which inevitably leads to politics (with a small *p*). Religion or any other hierarchical organization involves the same.

The Tibetans believe that this manipulating is part of human nature; that in these sorts of situations, people come to believe that their activities and their emotions are the same. So they invest the energies of control into what they are doing and seek to stamp their personalities on it indelibly, so that other people will sit up and take notice of them.

This can be a good or a bad thing. In the end, however, the closer the identification becomes, the more likely it is that work itself becomes the obstruction. Eventually, it prevents the individual from becoming balanced.

The answer is this. If you are taking a position in any organization, do the following: know where the power comes from and who holds it, discover who holds all the emotional energy in your work community, and observe how the power holder and the emotion holder affect everyone else. Then, see if you want to be part of it.

3. Money: How It Is Made, Kept, and Used

Contrary to popular belief, you can take your money with you when you die. How? Most people are emotionally attached to their cash, and during life, this emotional attachment is actually more important than the cash. The same energy occupies the dying person's consciousness.

Of itself, money is invisible. Sure, there are bills, coins, checks, and credit cards, but all of these are simply representations of money. Money is, and has always been, an agreement of value and a symbol of trust.

The energy of money is like the wind, invisible but felt all around the world. It is an aspect of humankind's higher thought made manifest in the material world.

Money is a mirror into which few people have the courage to look, but doing so can help you to attract large amounts of cash. Remembering that money is a process of thought and energy, start by sensing the energy of money in the everyday world around you. Notice the way money influences your life, your culture, and the development of your country and the global community.

Now look at how you make your living. This must be in accordance with what makes you happy. Many people make lots of money from occupations that do not make them happy, and then, like a time bomb, there comes a point when their money becomes an obstruction in itself. They lose it by one means or another—devaluation, taxation, or bad advice. Then, making money suddenly loses its allure.

The ancient Tibetan approach to attracting and keeping money is simple. Remember that money is energy, so you need to balance it. Remember that cash, credit cards, stocks, debts, and bills are merely symbols of this energy. Remember, too, that although this energy can be stern and unforgiving, you have the power to change that.

Now meditate on this energy by focusing for a few minutes once a day on all your financial assets, big or small. Concentrate on them one by one and send them positive thoughts, telling them to increase and multiply so that they benefit you and others.

Remember that in today's world, your bank account, for example, is not a solitary financial island but is connected to other financial systems, so the money energy that flows throughout the world flows also through your bank account.

As you understand this connection, you will be able to send your mental energy out from your financial island. Imagine your energy as a big ship sailing worldwide, bringing back financial abundance to your island and also dropping off blessings to other islands throughout its voyage.

Always give what you can afford to those who are less fortunate than you. Money energy that is surplus should be shared, not stored. Wealth is what money can do for you in regard to other people. If this energy is abused, it seeks retribution and does not stay long with a mean master.

4. Health: How to Create It, Keep It, and Use It

Like money, health is an energy that must be balanced, looked after, and used wisely. The simplest way to care for your health is to respect your body, your mind, your speech, and your thoughts, as I describe in this book. You are not a commodity. You are a highly refined consciousness in a physical form. You are sacred.

5. Good Fortune: How to Make It, Keep It, and Use It

Good fortune comes about when the energies of your body and your mind click together. This is not just about the creation of wealth: Good fortune is the experience of knowing deep inside you that everything is right with the world. It is when you and the divine enjoy each other's company.

Good fortune is a natural state of mind that is part of who you are. It is inside you, just waiting to be released. Start by asking for it. Be humble and receive. If you seek good fortune unskillfully—in other words, selfishly—you will create obstructions.

It never comes in the way you expect it, so open your heart for a happy surprise. You keep your good fortune by sharing it and learning from it, not by showing it off. Use your good fortune by showing other people how to access theirs, based on your experience.

6. Repetitive Obstructions:
Why Problems Keep Coming Back

Obstructions that return repeatedly do so because they have not been healed. They are also trying to tell you how to deal with the problem. The answer to an obstruction always lies in the problem itself.

First, look at the history. When did the problems first start? Think back to when they occurred and focus on that moment; then you will discover the seed of the obstruction and its nature. Send it as much love as you can. This will start to transform the obstruction into a problem with the potential for change.

Obstructions can seem insurmountable, but, by directing love to them, they are acknowledged and start to reveal what they are made of. In this way, they lose their intensity and weight until finally the essence of the problem is revealed.

Imagine, for instance, that someone is in constant debt, which he never manages to repay. In his mind, the obstruction set up by this situation has grown more powerful than the actual debt and the obligation to pay it. So, the person is unable to confront the original problem.

By directing love to this situation, however, the obstruction dissolves and the debtor creates inner distance and a new perspective on the problem. As this happens, the obstruction shows the individual how to heal it once and for all. Then, the debtor works out a way of paying what is owed, and understands how to avoid getting in that situation again.

7. Family and Friends

There are two families in your life: the family you are born to and the family you make—that is, your friends. Your relationship with your birth family influences how you make and value friendships. If you have problems with family or friends, you need to start to understand the way in which the problem affects you and others.

Look at how you talk to each other—the language you all use, the type of words you use to express emotions. If you use harsh or swear words to express what you feel, you will only separate the opportunities for healing. Gentle words that are firm and direct, and questions that need responses, are better.

People choose harsh words because they are unsure of what they really want to say. Using lots of emotionally loaded words with open-ended questions is the same. A sentence such as, "Damn you, you never pay attention to what I say," may express how you feel, but it also places an energetic affliction on the person to whom you say it. So it is also important to listen to what others say with your heart and your mind, not just with your reactive emotions.

As you explore this, you will become aware of the emotional forces at the heart of most communication and can understand what people really mean. You start to see how obstructions occur and how they influence your life and the lives of your family and friends. Once this takes place, you are able to start a process of honest communication.

But changing yourself may be all that you can do. Your friends and family may not truly want to communicate from the heart. They may not even want honesty. Remember, it's up to them.

8. Spiritual Needs

Most people go through life firmly avoiding their spiritual needs. However, it is vital to consider this area. You may find that what you need is vastly different from what you imagined. The first step is to be prepared to recognize that you do not know anything at all. This is tough! But after the mental shock of accepting this has passed, you understand that you are more than your name, body, reputation, bank balance, and desires. All of these cover up your inner spiritual consciousness, and it is this internal knowledge that shows you what you truly are and what you truly know.

Often we embark on things in life that we believe are important—a job, say, a campaign or a relationship—only to discover that they did not satisfy us in the way we had expected. This is because nothing that is external to us can deliver the satisfaction that our everyday minds hope for. We forget that all we need to find satisfaction in our lives is to connect with our inner selves and to understand that spirituality exists in everything we do.

The inner self speaks to us continously, but often the everyday mind cannot recognize the words. Our inner wisdom knows that everything in the everyday world has a spiritual essence. Spiritual growth starts with the most ordinary things you do each day, from cleaning the house to brushing your teeth. And it is through these mundane activities that you will find your inner divinity, not through your job title, bank balance, or relationships.

9. Right Actions, Skillful Thoughts

Right actions come from skillful or right thinking. Right action means doing what is right for you and for other people; it also means taking responsibility for your actions.

Skillful thinking is a process that enables you to be happy, focused, and calm, and, in this way, it supports your actions. Skillful thoughts also help you to come to an understanding of your inner morality and ethical framework, so understanding your spiritual needs is vital. This is an individual thing, differing from person to person. The ancient Tibetans believed that although society and religious beliefs should have basic rules and guidelines, each person must find his or her own morality and ethics. This is the foundation for emotional and spiritual maturity.

10. Creating Good Energy

By focusing on these areas of your life, you will see the nature of the problems and obstructions that are common to virtually everyone on this planet. Simply starting the process of changing them will help to cultivate stronger mental energies. All you need is to be willing to try.

At times in our lives, we may come across obstructions that are so powerful, the only way to transform the situation is to accept it with humility and grace. Then you will be able to see the spiritual significance of why the problem can be changed only in this way.

At times, you can change your circumstances only by embracing the spiritual within you.

These ten insights into obstructions can be understood and overcome by using the ten ways to create well-being. For every problem that you encounter, the following techniques will show you how to turn things around.

Ten Ways to Create Well-being

These ten ways come from a section of Tibetan Bön teachings known as The Way of the Shen of the Cha. They can be used as a form of internal divination to help you increase the quality and quantity of your happiness, improve your vitality, and be more successful in all your chosen activities.

Each way is accompanied by a traditional action on which to focus, which stimulates the mind and the body. I have adapted some of them slightly so that they make sense in our modern world. However, the content of each way stems from ancient Tibetan wisdom that has been refined over thousands of years.

Each way is a channel that can direct your experience from within you and out into the world. You can use any of the ten ways that seem most relevant, or you can use all ten over a ten-day period. If you are attracted to a particular way, do it for ten days at the same time each day.

These ten ways of thought and action are useful tools for creating mental and emotional awareness in how you conduct your daily life. They introduce you gently to a new reality, which is often quite different from the version you are currently occupying. They are tools for living the life you want, and for acquiring power and wisdom.

Expect results as soon as you start.

The First Way

Treating your illness with kindness will encourage faster recovery or resolution. You will gain a stronger mental approach to life so that you can direct your actions in accordance with your aims.

THE ACTION

Imagine a seed starting to grow from the earth. Watch it turn into a beautiful tree with pink flowers and golden fruit. The flowers have a most beautiful smell and the fruit is sweet and juicy. Smell the flowers so that you become the perfume. Eat the fruit so that you become the taste. Some of the flowers and fruit fall to the earth, and as the tree dies, a new one grows exactly as before.

The Second Way

Dwell upon those aspects of your life that can be improved. As you take the action below, you will gain deep insight into the qualities of your potential.

THE ACTION

A fragile golden bell sways with the wind. It is suspended by a red and gold thread covered with little knots hung across a round brass frame. You pick up a long, delicate silver hammer from a red cushion. The hammer head is in the shape of an elephant with a raised trunk. At the end is a perfectly shaped sphere covered with engraved flower petals. You breathe in and out slowly, then gently strike the bell. The tone of the bell is soft at first, then grows like a beautiful voice within you. Your mind becomes clear.

The Third Way

If you want to overcome the energies of anger, lust, and greed, you need to understand how you created them and gave them life.

THE ACTION

What anger, lust, and greed want most of all is recognition. Think of them as three unruly children who mimic everything you say and do. Shouting at them to stop does nothing. Anger is dressed in black clothes, lust in red, greed in green. Acknowledge them, asking each one by name what it wants to say and what it is trying to tell you. Listen carefully and with humility. You will get a reply, although it may not be to your liking at first. As they speak, give them as much love as they can receive. This will forever change them and you for the better.

The Fourth Way

You are not a slave to life. Life is a mountain range through which you can navigate using your internal direction finder, which comes from developing discernment and discretion.

THE ACTION

In front of you are three bowls, one full of diamonds, the second emeralds, and the third rubies. As you watch them, the bowls and their precious contents merge into one unit. In your mind's eye, start to separate them bowl by bowl, jewel by jewel, until they are as they were before.

The Fifth Way

Become aware of how and where your body stores stress and negativity. By knowing this, you can stop this process.

THE ACTION

Imagine that you are lying on your back, stretched out and at ease. A violet light appears over your head and starts to flow down your body, fading as it passes over your feet. You feel warm. Slowly, patches of black and of gray appear over your body where you feel most stressed and anxious. In the areas of black, focus a gold light to release stress from your physical body. In the areas of gray, focus a pink light to release stress from your mental body.

The Sixth Way

Perhaps you suspect that your job is making you ill, bringing out one side of your personality at the expense of other aspects of your life. If so, this is creating unneeded negativity that will diminish your mind and body and your happiness.

THE ACTION

Contemplate this image: A man (or a woman) works all day long to provide the best for the family. Then he starts to work at night, too. He becomes so obsessed by the emotional attachment to his work that he doesn't notice that he has grown apart from his spouse and family. Suddenly he loses his job. He has no work and no connection to his family. This individual now has nothing.

This nothing is the best possession anyone could ever have. The person discovers that he is not his job. We can all create employment by knowing who we are and who we have the potential to be. This is also true for our families.

This situation happens every day all over the world. It is part of human nature, but it can be changed.

The Seventh Way

Examine how your food and drink affect your mood and the way your body responds. This will show you what foods are best for you and how your mind affects the food you have eaten.

THE ACTION

Treat everything you eat and drink with respect, whether it is health food, home cooking, restaurant fare, or junk food. What matters is not what you eat but how you eat it. Your attitude creates the effects your food has on your body and mind and therefore your attitude to the way you live and regard other people. Eating with respect is the same as praying. Food is prayer in action. Every morsel is an exercise in consciousness.

The Eighth Way

Every time we speak, we change other people's lives. Be aware of what you say, of the thought processes behind it, and its influence on others.

THE ACTION

Repeat this slowly, out loud, word by word:

What is the most potent weapon in the history of humankind? Forget terrorism, nuclear bombs, napalm, and biological weapons, although they are all horrific. The greatest weapon is the human tongue and the way it is used. Speech is the action of thought; it affects people's lives in subtle ways, often forever. When you insult others, you insult yourself. Genuine praise or other forms of compassionate or honorable language, however, act as gifts. They can bring humility to the speaker and insight and power to the listener. Speech is one of humankind's greatest achievements because it comes from the desire to communicate truth and share common feelings. Do not let your speech be taken for granted by others or yourself. It is not a commodity but a sacred event. Often it is better to be silent than to say something foolish. Silence teaches us the value of language. May peace be upon me and upon the world.

The Ninth Way

Activate your inner truth and your own morality by allowing yourself to be as good as you can. Life is a series of emotional and intellectual constructions—the architecture of the mind. If you understand how your mind influences all aspects of your life, you will become less reactive to life's difficulties.

THE ACTION
Take ten minutes a day to be silent. Listen to your thoughts. Use your inner senses to see what they are made of. See what is important to your life and which activities detract from your sense of goodness. This is not easy, but it is worthwhile. You will be surprised at how much goodness lies inside you waiting to be used. As you connect to your goodness, you become still and more focused; you are less easily distracted by events, actions of life, and other people's thoughts and desires. This starts to create a foundation for wisdom. Your wisdom is your power.

The Tenth Way

Give thanks for the good times and the bad. Forgive all those who have hurt you and ask for forgiveness for yourself.

THE ACTION

Imagine you have thousands of beautiful white flowers, each with a different perfume. Smell each one very slowly, putting your attention into each bloom. In front of you is a fire in a triangular hearth, painted in yellow and red triangular patterns, with the point of the triangle pointing away from you. Put your attention into the fire. Now pick up one flower at a time and think of a hurt, or a state of anger, lust, greed, or hate that was sparked by an action taken by you or someone else.

Say aloud the name of the person you are thinking of, or describe the situation, and thank him or her three times, whether the experience was good or bad. This helps you to let go of the past, of pain, and of the cycle of suffering. It also stops dangerous and other bad situations from becoming worse.

Put the emotion of these negative experiences into a flower and then place it into the fire. Watch the flower burn. Do this with each flower until they are all gone. Say again the name of the person or description of the situation, and again give your thanks. This will help to terminate the particular cycle of suffering. The past will lose its sting.

At the end of this chapter, there are three very important points to remember. Just as the ten insights into obstructions are directives for action, so these three simple points can be seen as mental stepping-stones on your path to a balanced and wise life.

1. Illness and health come from the same inner workings of your mind. All aspects of the material world, including your thoughts, are created by how you view reality.

2. As an individual, you are made up of five threads of mental energy. Your mind fabricates these in order to

make sense of the world. They are: awareness, acceptance, determination, discernment, and attachment. These five threads weave themselves into all human activity.

Awareness enables you to understand how you come to suffer and what your true needs are.

Acceptance of your circumstances and situations that you cannot change (principally, other people) makes you aware of karma and brings compassion.

Determination helps you to overcome all obstacles.

Discernment helps you to find the essence and truth of all things.

Attachment is the thread around which the other four are wrapped. By knowing how you are attached to things, and why, you become less attached and begin to know what is truly important to you in your life.

3. Regardless of your actions and thoughts, you, like everyone else, originated from the energy of fundamental goodness. Life's experiences can make you forget this, which causes pain. To be as good as you know how is the first and last medicine, which will, in time, heal all things.

CHAPTER SEVEN

Recovery and Rejuvenation

Healing is all about rejuvenation. It is your right. Take it and use it for your own benefit and for the benefit of everyone else, too. Learning the process of rejuvenation is easy because the innate ability to do so is within you at every level.

The wisdom in this chapter will help you to get the most out of your life and to discover the essence of living. You will discover the theory of the five elements that make up everything in the universe, how to use this knowledge in a series of self-healing exercises, how to make friends with your body, and how to achieve high energy, deep focus, and lasting concentration.

Being ill is a difficult experience. As you discovered in chapter 6, Tibetan medicine looks at the foundations of illness and the path to healing in this way: People suffer and get ill, both physically and emotionally, through ignorance of the appropriate way to create well-being. If they have the right means to cure their suffering, however, illness can become health and balance.

In order to help yourself get well and stay well, you need to go to the original influence that made you ill and heal it. Then your body, mind, and life will start to rejuvenate. You will feel as if you have been reborn. You will be younger in mind, spirit, and body. The process of aging will slow down and your wisdom will increase.

GETTING WELL ...

First, let us consider the basic steps of recovery that we all go through when regaining well-being, whether the illness is physical, emotional, mental, or spiritual.

- Recovery: The process of becoming stable when your mind and body are no longer adversely affected by sickness.

- Renewal: When your body and mind start to repair and you are no longer sick.

... AND STAYING WELL

This is the step that we need to take if we want true health.

- Rejuvenation: When you discover the underlying cause of your condition through a mental or spiritual process so that both your life and your state of mind are totally transformed.

Rejuvenation is an attitude of mind, a statement of consciousness, and a physical process. It is your physical body transforming itself into a higher physical state. This is joyful and powerful. And it lasts forever. Even though your body will die at some point, the experience of rejuvenation will live on in your soul and the souls of others.

Rejuvenation renews your senses, body, brain, intellect, and emotions. As you experience heightened vitality, mental clarity, and spiritual integration, you empower your soul and gain self-knowledge.

All of us need to discover the knowledge to rejuvenate but some people are more obviously in need than others. Perhaps you have had to communicate with or look after someone who is very ill or in constant pain, terminally ill, or seriously injured. You may sense that he seems dormant. His breathing does not seem to give him life, to inspire him. You often notice the same thing with people who always seem to be sick with chronic complaints such as colds, aches and pains, sore bones, or headaches.

For these people, illness has become a routine that is essential to their lives. They need their problems and have lost their true selves in them. Such people need to recover, renew, and rejuvenate. The means to do so are contained within the theory of the five elements.

The Five Elements

All things in this world and in the cosmos at large, including your body and mind, are in a state of intertwining flux and form. These forces seem powerful, valid, and real but in fact they are fleeting and impermanent, in a continuous process of change. Every aspect of thought and belief, of the physical world and of the universe, is born, has its time, dies, and is recycled again into energy. The weavers of this vast tapestry are, according to Tibetan belief, the five elements—Earth, Water, Fire, Wind/Air, and Space.

The influence of the five elements defines the universe and the laws of nature, including the energetic relationships of your mind and body. This means that everything in the material world, great and small, starts and finishes with the elements. They are also intrinsically connected to our health through the three humors—Wind, Bile, and Phlegm—which you discovered in the preceding chapter. Knowing the five elements and how they work with the three humors can enable you to understand your place in the material world.

The nature of the five elements is hard for the Western mind to accept. They are simultaneously symbolic, descriptive, subjective, and actual. Confusingly, they do not always refer literally to the physical elements after which they are named, but this need not concern you now. They are the energies that make all things work, from the universe to the solar system, from lunar influences to the world at large, from your nation to your city and community and, of course, your body.

The five elements are crucial to health because they are the basic ingredients for the origins and the cures of disease. The qualities of each element are aspects of our consciousness. Each creates deep-seated structures that support our unconscious minds and our instinctual drives and intuition. They form the way we view ourselves and build our personalities.

When the elements are out of balance in your life, things may not work the way you want them to. By balancing the elements, you experience a spontaneous understanding of them and an awareness of the energies of the natural world. Then you begin to gain great insight into the nature of your personality, releasing huge amounts of energy that you can use to benefit yourself and others.

We can harness the potential of the five elements to help us by using meditations that incorporate visualization. These are detailed later. Don't worry if you find it hard to picture things in your mind; just following the instructions will bring good results.

Earth

Earth is the material nature of things: matter, weight, durability, and density. It rules the structure of our bodies—the musculoskeletal system—and the way we respond to our surroundings.

This element is involved in creating all types of muscle in the body, all aspects of bone development, bone marrow, and the growth of skin, eyes, and their functions. It influences smell and also the way in which our physical senses interact with one another. Earth also awakens our perceptions of time and the experiences of daily living, death, and birth.

The Earth element connects us to the underlying rhythms of our health and shows us what we can learn from becoming ill and the wisdom to be gained within that. It reflects our consciousness and shows us who we really are, reminding us of our physical impermanence.

Earth provides stability, direction, discipline, and tolerance.

Water

Water influences the composition of our bodies and our emotional needs. It is essentially the lubricating generative force that unites the merging of matter between the subatomic world and the cellular one. In our bodies, water is the cohesive factor driving all the major systems.

This element is involved in creating all aspects of body fluids, from urine, lymph, and blood to all types of discharges, both internal and external. Water directs taste and its process within the body. It influences how we become ill and the effects of those illnesses, and gives us energy to prevent us from becoming ill. This element influences religious thought, emotions, changes in human history, and the development of faith.

Water creates fluid thought, compassion, intuitive and empathic qualities, humility, and generosity.

Fire

Fire influences and directs the health of the body and mind. It is the evolution and growth of matter; within the body it is heat, digestive functions, and the spark within the regulatory systems of the metabolism.

The Fire element helps strengthen the immune system, the body's defense against illness. It controls body temperature, influences circulation and heart function, and vision. Fire can show us why we get ill and how all things in the body become disconnected when one part is sick. It influences the worlds of money, business, and career.

Fire creates the desire for overcoming obstructions and for self-development, inspiration, wisdom, and joy.

Wind/Air

Wind/Air is the powerful moving force that influences oxygenation and circulatory, pulmonary, neural, and lymphatic activity. It sparks cardiac function, influencing heart chambers to pump, while it regulates brain function, creating the invisible link between mind, personality, and body function. Wind/Air creates the way in which we react to other people.

Wind/Air controls and directs breathing and all metabolic aspects of respiration. It governs the functions of the body's organs. Because it influences touch, Wind/Air helps you—unconsciously—to have a greater knowledge of your immediate environment. It also influences academic thought and discipline.

Wind/Air creates an inquiring mind, love of knowledge and reasoning, respect for community, and the desire for freedom.

Space

Space is the underlying element that forms the development of our physical and mental personalities. It allows the dynamic interplay of the other elements. This element creates all spaces, orifices, and cavities in every part of your physical body and your mind; it is our potential for expanded awareness. It also influences the ability to think creatively.

This element influences your hearing and everything associated with it; for example, hearing good news or bad, or listening to gossip. Space is the potential for consciousness to be evolved and liberated; it reveals the highest in all human nature.

Exploring the concept of elemental Space can reveal to us how and why we make ourselves sick and help us to activate rejuvenation.

How to Understand and Use Your Elemental Nature

At the start or end of each season, you can begin to gain insight into your elemental nature simply by watching the seasonal change. You can also tune in to the moon when it is either full or new, looking at it and allowing your senses to feel it. As you do this, focus on the elements one by one. You will sense them within you. Start to feel which are more dominant and which are weak.

As you look at the natural world, note the correspondences between the elements. Then, examine your personality and see how it relates to the elements in nature that attract you the most.

Draw a circle on a large piece of paper. Divide the circumference of the circle into five equal sections. Above each section write in the name of one of the five elements. Use a different color for each—choose ones that you think match them. Then write in your feelings about each element. You will slowly begin to build up a personal elemental circle and be able to see which ones are balanced and which are not.

The more you do this simple exercise, the more you will start to stimulate deep unconscious pathways between your everyday mind and the elements. Creating this circle will also start to show you which of your habits are fueled by a particular element and help you to gain insight into how to improve things.

ELEMENTAL IMBALANCES

These are caused by emotional negativity. If we cannot understand that we are the cause of our suffering and we blame our problems on external events, the negativity will increase, strengthening the elemental imbalances even more.

If we become used to perceiving only suffering or bad experiences, we create mental pain for ourselves. When we focus unskillfully on the cause of our unhappiness—or endlessly question our right to happiness—the experience intensifies until it is bound to collapse, causing us further unhappiness and disrupting our elemental harmony. Then, whatever we experience—good or bad—we treat with suspicion. That's a great shame because it means we lose connection with our inherent openness and innocence.

USING THE FIVE ELEMENTS TO ACTIVATE REJUVENATION

Genuine, lasting change can happen only if you transmute the patterns in your life that cause you illness or recurring pain.

This means becoming a more balanced person than you were before you became sick. You need to identify how your body stores pain, reacts to it, and then expresses it.

We can use the five elements to help us. Each of them is a key to knowing about the story of your body. Crucially, in order to change, you need to feel that within you there is the space or emotional room for this to happen.

If you are finding it hard to bend your mind to instigate the first steps of rejuvenation, the problem is that the Phlegm humor is restricting the possibilities of growth and change. The following self-healing exercise will help to transform your thought patterns and heal blocked emotions. It combines the skillful use of Fire (motivation), Wind/Air (movement), and Space (the possibility of change).

Self-Healing Exercise 1

This will help to heal blocked emotions and stimulate change.

Sit or lie down comfortably. Focus on your breathing.

With your mind and breath, start to try and feel all the cavities in your body. Take your time. Feel the shapes of the cavities and orifices of your body, including your mouth, sinuses, bladder, stomach, intestines, and ears. You can also explore the cavities in your joints, nostrils, eye sockets, etc.

Use your breath to gain a sense of the size and depth of these cavities. Once you can do this, let your mind fill those spaces. Then imagine all of them merging into one.

Feel the element of Wind/Air flow through this larger space, all through your body, into your bones. Move, clear, and clean any and all types of obstructions, both physical and mental.

Your desire for change starts to unfold as a feeling of physical strength. Your body becomes relaxed and feels stretched out.

At this point, you feel your bodily cavities start to generate heat. Slowly, a gentle fire begins to emanate from the spaces, warming your whole body, flowing through your bloodstream, relaxing your muscles and bones and strengthening your desire to be free of illness.

Let your body rest in this warmth and start to see yourself becoming well and going about your life filled with power, joy, and strength.

Do this exercise slowly, twice a day if you can, at home and at work, for thirteen days in a row. It will give you courage and help you to feel in control again, but in a new way. You will feel at home in your body.

Rachel had long-term chronic fatigue syndrome and regular attacks of severe asthma. Most of the time she was in bed, angry and ill. She felt completely powerless and trapped by her condition. She got to the stage of giving up trying to get well. So she got worse.

Then she decided to try Tibetan medicine. After a few months she felt a little better and was introduced to this self-healing exercise, which she used as part of her treatment. Her attitude became much more positive and within a year she was up and about. After another year, her asthma disappeared completely. She is now able to work, as a result of her treatment.

The exercise empowered Rachel to understand the nature of her physical suffering. "I felt powerless, out of control, and didn't know what to do. I gained a huge amount by using the meditation exercise, and became more connected. I am able to direct my own life now, instead of leaving it to doctors, parents, or friends. At last, I am truly independent."

REJUVENATION AND RECOVERY ARE NOT THE SAME

"Recovery is a valley, rejuvenation is a mountain," according to an old Tibetan saying. This means that you can get better without knowing why you were sick, which in turn means that you can become ill again. Rejuvenation is the total renewal of mind and body, so that from the mountain peak you have a complete view of the valley and can detect all the complexities of the landscape.

Sickness is not greater than you; it is part of you, defined by your experience of living. To have the full picture of your sickness means you can decide to have power over whatever ails or influences you and can then determine the outcome.

It is important to understand that your inner mind goes through the rejuvenation experience first. Then, like a flash of bright light, it floods the physical body with energizing and healing power. All of this is latent within you, a submerged frequency of energy waiting to be used.

The process is called a *jinlab*, or "wave of grace," in Tibetan, a moment of spiritual beauty that is both ascending and descending. You can receive this blessing from others, but you can also give it to yourself.

Charles had motor neuron disease. He knew he was near death and was terrified of dying painfully by suffocation. He came to believe that nothing could change his illness, that in some way he was being "punished" for whatever bad things he had done in the past. As his body let him down, he felt more powerless by the day.

Charles had been famous all over the world for half a century, but he knew his fame could do nothing to help him. At this nadir, he was introduced to the notion of rejuvenation instead of recovery.

167

*At first he didn't see the point of doing the self-healing
exercise, but finally he understood that it could ease his fear
of dying. In fact, it rejuvenated his inner life, and when he
died a few weeks later, he had no fear.*

*"Overcoming my fear of death showed me not to be afraid
of life," he told me moments before he died. "I know why I
got sick. Now I am rejuvenated. I am ready."*

At his funeral, his wife sang "Amazing Grace."

Self-Healing Exercise 2

This will help heal the fear of dying, both for the person and
caregivers, friends, and family. It also calms those who are
frightened of success.

Focus on your heartbeat. Let its rhythms pulse through you
until all you sense and feel is your heartbeat. Feel the element
of Fire start to grow from a little flame, larger and larger. The
beat of your heart fans the fire of rejuvenation.

Now imagine that your skin begins to glow a light red. Your
body is full of this gentle fire. You start to sense the movement
and heat of powerful healing energies as the Bile humor
becomes active.

As this happens, the Earth element starts to be felt in your
skeleton, emerging as a powerful but gentle sensation spreading through your bones and joints, inflating your skeleton with
a strong, stable force.

Rest in this energy. Close your eyes and merge into it.

New Body, New Intelligence

Your body has its own innate ability to sense the environment
around it, and this unconsciously feeds into the way your mind
deals with the world. By activating the Wind/Air element and
the Wind humor, as described in self-healing exercise 3, you

can start to develop a connection with your body that gives you greater awareness of it and more-heightened senses. This establishes within you a truer sense of your physical reality and is a crucial part of the rejuvenation experience.

Malcolm suffered from a muscle-wasting disease, which conventional medicine was treating with a rigorous program of drugs and exercise. When he came to see me he was unhappy and isolated. He felt his body was an enemy, a slave master to which he was manacled. Since his teens he had wanted to be a professional tennis player, but his illness developed at much the same time and he had to give up his dream. Years of resentment against his body built up within him. Malcolm and his body did not have a good relationship. As he practiced this exercise, he began slowly to transform his anger and frustration and started to find new ways of appreciating his body, even enjoying it. Eventually he was able to create a marvelous state of self-love within. As a result of this dynamic and healthy mind-body relationship, he exudes charisma and compassion. "I don't hate myself anymore," he told me. "I feel like other people—normal."

Self-Healing Exercise 3

This will help you to enhance your connection with your body. Focus on your breathing. With your mind, tell the Wind/Air element to circulate throughout your body; it will automatically find its own course. Now focus on the Wind humor as it moves from the top of your head down into your pelvis. The more you do this exercise, the more you will be able to feel both the Wind/Air element and the Wind humor as they travel through you.

They automatically stimulate the Earth element and your body starts to inflate with power. At the same time, the Air element helps your body to feel calm and flowing.

Relax. Be as still as you can. Let the energy of the elements and the humors activate your body to expand and stretch. As you start to feel all the physical functions of the body becoming energized and flexible, your mind merges with your body and they are one.

Be still.

ILLNESS IS COMMUNICATION

Becoming ill is the desperate stage in communication at which your body and mind announce war on you. Emotional and physical processes under stress strive to be expressed in a form that makes you sit up and take notice. The body and the soul use a language of immediate experiences that remind us of our mortality and fragility. And it can take place at any time, anywhere.

> Despite being a leading academic, Harry never paid attention to his body. After many decades of this neglect, he ended up with illnesses ranging from liver and kidney disease to late-onset diabetes. He was overwhelmed and could make no sense of what was happening to him. He felt that he had "no space inside [his] head or his body."
>
> Harry decided to escape. He gave up his prestigious job at a famous American university and moved to London. But he soon discovered that his problems had traveled with him.
>
> Nothing improved significantly until he learned to use the self-healing exercise below to break free of his confusion and allow him to listen to his body. Then he heard the clear words of health underneath the troubled buzz of sickness. He returned to America and went through a course of treatment.
>
> Eventually he learned how to manage both his body and his mind. Harry went back to work and became happy.

Self-Healing Exercise 4

This will help you to confront your fears.

Lie straight, if possible, or sit comfortably with your hands resting in your lap. Close your eyes.

Focus on your skeleton. Feel it. Imagine the Water element flowing through each bone, a pipe of life. Let your mind flow with the Water in your bones. Feel its power. Let your mind allow the Water element to focus your attention.

Follow the flow until you come to rest naturally.

There Is No Room for Habits That Restrict Rejuvenation

Negative patterns of behavior, such as chain-smoking, taking drugs, and obsessional attitudes, can restrict your physical well-being and sow the seeds of illness. By knowing what is good for you and what is not, you can implement rejuvenation.

Michael, a musician, got into the habit of being sick as a means of coping with stress, fatigue, and fame. He did everything he could to sabotage his understanding of why he was ill. When he learned this self-healing exercise, he began to admit to himself that he had to give up the habits that supported his illnesses.

Step by step, this inner awareness evolved into Michael's knowing what was good for him. He started to discover a yearning for spirituality and to feel a desire for happiness. He let go of his addiction to his career and the fame that came with it and was then able to take charge. His music improved and so did his record sales. So did his happiness. He no longer isolates himself, but takes a full part in his community.

Self-Healing Exercise 5

This will help to heal addiction of any type and enhance the ability to see through self-created illusions.

Lie on your back. Focus on your belly, the source of physical power. Follow the rise and fall of your breathing.

In the depth of your gut, try to feel your Water element moving through the tissues of your muscles and skin. Feel the coolness of this Water running over your skin.

Now activate your Wind humor: Simply think of it and feel it spiraling up from your groin, fanning out to the top of your head and taking with it the negativity and physical poisons. As this happens, imagine the Wind humor becoming an orange light that removes and destroys all the pollution in your mind and body.

Rest quietly for a few moments, just feeling the state of your body and mind.

YOUR INTELLIGENT BODY

Whatever you think, do, or experience profoundly influences your body, as does every aspect of your physical world. It absorbs all experiences and places them within your nervous system, which then creates your immediate reality.

Your mind, however, can be tricked by sensory influences, language, and belief systems. It believes what it receives. But the body believes only what it can use. It stores pain, for instance, as part of its learning process.

The problem is that your body often doesn't have the means to distinguish what to keep and what to let go. Helping it to do so is a vital key to rejuvenation. You can then determine the way in which your body deals with illness and help it to create well-being.

Matthew was always tired and in pain and had little energy for anything. His body seemed out of control and separate from his mind—he felt he was losing connection with it.

Little experiences in his daily life escalated into major dramas, so that by the time he went to bed he was so tired he couldn't sleep. His body had become confused by what was happening in the world around it.

He was prescribed Tibetan herbal medicine and a program of Kum Nye exercises. When he learned the self-healing exercise below, he began to understand that he was suffering from an acute stress disorder. The exercise allowed him to discover a way of creating emotional boundaries through which he could interpret the world safely.

Based on what he learned, Michael changed his life-style and was able to cure himself completely.

Self-Healing Exercise 6

This will help you to unlock your healing abilities.

Lie down on your back or sit comfortably, hands in lap, eyes closed.

Sense your skeleton, feeling the large bones in your legs and the long bones in your arms. Feel the length of your spine and the top and back of your head. Place your sensations of these areas into your general awareness by breathing through them and letting go of any tensions.

Feel the natural connection between these areas as the energy you release seeks to move through your body. Now direct the energy back into your spine, moving from the top of your neck down through each vertebrae to the base of your spine.

Rest, and focus on your physical heart. Receive what your heart tells you. That might be feelings or emotions, physical sensations such as pain, memories, happiness, even a recipe for pie. Anything. Just receive what comes.

REPAIR, RESTORE, REJUVENATE: YOU CAN DO IT!

Your body wants to grow, renew, expand, rejuvenate, and survive, but it is always timid about the healing process. It needs to be encouraged like a shy child.

Cultivating positive thought is vital to the body's learning to stay well. You can use the fact that the body forgets nothing. Once a thought is properly placed, the body keeps it to continue to a higher state of survival.

Self-Healing Exercise 7

This will help you to have the courage to accept those things you cannot change.

Lie down on your back or sit comfortably, hands in lap, eyes closed.

Now think of the Water element flowing through your body.

As you do so, focus on how your body responds when you become sick, and on whether you really view your life in a positive way. You will find that you start to remember how your body responds when you are ill.

Send the Water element like a flowing stream through your skeleton, washing away all impurities. Then do the same for all your muscles and organs, including your skin. Think of sparkling drops of silver rain falling on and through you, warm and electric, renewing you from the inside out. As this silver rain falls on you, start to breathe it in.

Feel the vitality surging throughout your body.

Loving Energy Is in Everything

Whatever your circumstances, your immediate surroundings contain boundless positive energy.

According to Tibetan medicine, matter is slow-moving energy, and your consciousness can make any matter relax, open, and become pliable. You can make it speed up or slow down. The energy in your surroundings is like a golden cup covered with grime, which your mind can clean so that it shines with love and positivity.

Self-Healing Exercise 8

This will help you to experience love in all things.

Lie down on your back or sit comfortably, hands in lap, eyes closed.

Focus on your breathing. As you breathe in and out slowly and deeply, focus on the five elements—Space, Wind/Air, Fire, Water, and Earth—around you. Feel each growing in powerful healing energy with every breath you take.

As you do so, the energy of the elements in your surroundings will start to be drawn toward you. As you feel this happening, focus on your heart and see a deep emerald-green light shining there. The five elements flow into this light and filter into your body for immediate healing and use.

Rest, and receive the energy. When you feel you cannot absorb any more, start to direct it out to all of your friends and enemies, to negative and positive situations and events, and to all living creatures so that they may benefit as you have.

Using Your Body's Inner Cycle

The Tibetans believe that the material world, the universe, and the mind go through cycles of rejuvenation. By working with the cycles, you unlock within yourself the basis of rejuvenation. You can use your body's inner cycle by this self-healing exercise.

Self-Healing Exercise 9

This will help you to understand the cycles of life and know that there is an appropriate time for all things to happen.

Stretch out on your back, with both arms and legs slightly apart. Become aware of your breathing, then your heartbeat.

Let your Wind/Air and Water elements become active. Just think about each one and in your mind say its name. Close your eyes to help you to concentrate. As you do so, you will discover—underneath the movement of your breathing and your heartbeat—other physical cycles and functions in your body.

Follow each one and you will feel it working in harmony with the next, like an orchestra. Timing, rhythm, and balance are the health gifts of the body's inner cycles.

Rejuvenation Is a Pattern

Throughout the natural world there are patterns that reveal the flux and flow of life force. Look at the patterns birds make when they fly in formation, the trails of clouds, the shapes that rivers carve through the landscape as they flow to the sea. Examine the minute detail of flowers and their petals, of seashells, of the five-pointed star at the core of an apple sliced sideways. Once you start looking at these, you will also see the intrinsic patterns of birth, death, and rejuvenation.

We human beings are as much a part of nature as flowers, sea creatures and apples, as the clouds, rivers, and birds. Exactly the same patterns exist within our bodies and our lives. Your body is the universe and the natural world in miniature. Think of the constant death and renewal of your skin cells every three or four weeks, of your bone cells every two years. As they course around your body, blood cells form a pattern very like flocks of migrating birds, and the sound of blood in your heart is exactly like waves on the seashore.

You can connect with the patterns of the natural world and feel the energy of life as the ancient Tibetans did, using a practice they called sky gazing. Simply gaze up into the heavens—blue, gray, thundery, day, or night—and let your mind soar up into the expanse. Feel its immensity. Free-float around the universe. Connect with the natural world.

DON'T JUDGE YOUR BODY, MAKE FRIENDS WITH IT

We all tend to judge ourselves by the way we look, how fit we are, and how much our bodies can or can't do. Nourishing a positive body image is crucial in the larger picture of well-being, but even that may slow down the rejuvenation process.

Whether you are vain about your body or disgusted by it, the result is the same—obsession. The best image you can cultivate about your body comes through listening to it and taking care of it. Your body's true value is far greater than you could ever conceive.

Self-Healing Exercise 10

This helps to show you just how precious your life is.

Lie down on your back or sit comfortably, hands in lap, eyes closed. Breathe gently and think about the marvel that is your body.

Let your mind remember for at least twenty minutes the

experiences gained from doing the exercises. Now focus again on your body and you will discover a shift in your consciousness as the rejuvenation process comes alive.

Rest.

Rejuvenation Is a Blessing from Within

The greatest blessings that you can receive are those that come from yourself. This doesn't mean that they are not triggered by some external means: Very often something you hear or see—a smile, music, a glint of sunshine, a line of poetry—leads to a moment of expanding consciousness within you.

Learn to be receptive to this endless river of healing, where you and the structures of the universe are intertwined in a fusion of consciousness. This is the nature of life, ever expanding and delighting in itself. Rejuvenation is a seed of energy that exists in the heart of even the most intense form of disease. You are that seed.

High Energy, Deep Focus, Lasting Concentration

High levels of mental and physical energy that enable you to focus deeply and with lasting concentration are a hugely desirable aspect of rejuvenation, but they can seem an impossible goal.

The ancient Tibetans regarded three qualities of energy, each influencing a different humor, as essential tools for self-knowledge and learning how to make the most of the world.

- High energy regulates and activates the Wind humor; it is a self-sustaining mental force that creates a well of inner energy to work effectively in the everyday world.

- Deep focus stimulates and balances Bile; it is creative energy that can be used to direct the outcome of the tasks you carry out.

- Lasting concentration regulates and integrates Phlegm; it brings you insight into how you live and conduct your personal affairs.

These three inner qualities can radically change your life for the better. By developing them through daily practice, you will enable yourself to become more active and clear-thinking. These powerful forces are available within you. All you need do is ask yourself whether you want them or not. If you do, read on. The meditation exercise on p. 184 will enable you to rediscover these essential qualities.

You may believe that you have never had any essential qualities that define who you really are. Everyone has. You have simply forgotten them or covered them up through life experiences. They can be awakened by transmuting your spiritual and emotional potential. Then you can use them in the everyday world.

These qualities may seem more worldly than spiritual. But, as with everything in the physical world, they integrate all aspects of living—mental, physical, emotional, and spiritual. Let us look at them in more detail.

High Energy

High energy will help you to work through problems, issues, or situations that seem insurmountable. This energy is everywhere; it is the building blocks of the molecular world and the foundation of light. It can be found in your physical heart and is perfectly active within you, seeking a harmonious connection with the material world where it can operate powerfully enough to overcome any and every type of obstruction.

Activating high energy will help you to be whole and strong, regardless of how you see yourself or your current circumstances. High energy develops within you compassion and the ability to stop yourself from repeating past mistakes, and helps to make your ideas become reality.

You will also be presented with many opportunities to create abundance and fame. This means you may have power or major influence over other people's lives. High energy enables you to be unattached to such things, while still using them skillfully. Developing this quality comes through a process of knowing why you are in the world and identifying your true role in life. You can also develop enduring joy, which is a quality of inner spiritual happiness that stays strong regardless of your circumstances.

Deep Focus

Deep focus comes from developing high energy. However, you need to know how to recognize, develop, and treasure it. Deep focus enables you to perceive the essence of anything and so to understand it. Understanding is power, and this kind of power helps you to become a better person. Being focused in this way encourages the ability to ask good questions on any subject and to cultivate the ability to discover quickly the truth of anything. This type of focus brings a deep appreciation of the spiritual in the commonplace.

Your mind will develop greater clarity and be able to remember large amounts of information. It will become disciplined, giving you the ability to think clearly. Deep focus also creates a respect for money and the ability to make, keep, and use it wisely.

Lasting Concentration

As your mind becomes more connected to your body and the world, lasting concentration rises like the morning sun, spreading its light and warmth. You begin to have a physical sensation of warmth and light.

This quality will empower you to gain the mental and emotional discipline needed to finish the things you start. It will also help you to bring together all types of activities, ideas, and experiences so that you can make sense of your world. The qualities of this form of concentration are the development of patience, faith, happiness, and enjoyment of the simple things in life. You are also more able to attract property, love, and general good fortune.

The Downsides of the Essential Qualities

As well as their beneficial aspects, each of the three qualities also has negative sides, which may cause damage at a later date. The qualities become negative only if people use them unskillfully.

- The negative qualities of high energy are: extreme vanity; self-obsession; paranoia; fear of flying or being enclosed in small spaces; addictions and addictive behaviors.

- The negative qualities of deep focus are: total exclusion of other people in the achievement of your aims; ruthless use of people or resources; anger over small things; the need to control; hoarding of resources; lack of generosity; violence toward others.

- The negative qualities of lasting concentration are: concern with detail to the exclusion of outcomes; meanness of spirit; rude behavior for no reason; jealousy; enjoyment in the suffering of others; a feeling of isolation from other people; inability to accept new ideas; a feeling that only bad things will happen or that there is no future happiness.

THE TEN CONNECTIONS

Before we go on to the meditation exercise, you will need to understand the mental connections necessary to activate and maintain the potential of these qualities. These concepts encourage your mind to accept the changes brought about by the meditation and integrate them into your personality. The connections will help you make sense of what you discover from the meditation.

1. Accept what you feel within yourself as you first start the meditation. Do not be afraid of the speed or intensity of the feelings that may emerge: This is a safe exercise.

2. Do not pay special attention to any images that come up in your mind or to any physical sensations that you feel while doing the meditation. These are responses from your body and mind to influences from the meditation.

3. Do not rush the exercise. Your mind and body will set their own pace. Your body will respond only at the speed that it feels is safe. Your mind is conditioned by your past mental attitudes and you cannot force it to respond immediately to inner change.

4. Mental and physical energy move at different rates. Your mind moves faster than your body because it is responding to millions of types of stimuli all at once.

Any changes that take place in the way your mind works will take a while to filter into your body. The meditation exercise will help to bring these two energies to a point where they will meet. You will intuitively feel the pace that they set. Do not try to force change; let it become a part of you naturally. If you can just sit back and let it come to you, you will benefit more.

5. You will make only as much progress as is appropriate. Be patient. Your mental energies will find their own balance naturally.

6. As you develop these qualities, they will bring out your mental abilities in a way that will surprise you. You may find latent resources that you never knew you had. Sometimes abilities about which you were insecure suddenly revive, and your former lack of confidence fades.

7. You will find a growing connection between your body and mind, unique to you. At first it will feel vague but in time it will become more definite. The more you practice this meditation, the more sensitive to each of the three qualities you will be, and the more intuitive about how they are affecting you.

8. Your mind will start to feel expanded and your body more relaxed. You will feel more alert and better able to carry out complicated mental tasks. These qualities will create a better mental state, and you will become more aware of how your mind works.

9. Your emotional energy will be calm. This means that the normal stresses of your everyday life will not affect you so intensely. You will know how to avoid creating further stress. This calmness will then grow and spread out into other aspects of your personality.

10. You will find that you have a more positive view about being alive. Courage, strength, fortitude, and direct behavior are aspects of this emerging positive energy.

MEDITATION EXERCISE TO ACTIVATE THE ESSENTIAL QUALITIES OF HIGH ENERGY, DEEP FOCUS, LASTING CONCENTRATION

Sit or lie down comfortably, eyes closed. Focus on your physical heart. Listen to its beating, its pulse. Allow this rhythm to flow through you.

Identify with your heartbeat. As you do so, think of your heartbeat becoming a milky-white light that flows over and through you. As you become infused with this light, all your fears and obstructions dissolve. The light becomes intense and more brilliant; it starts to make a flute-like sound. This washes over and through you until your personality and the workings of your mind become the same as the light and the sound.

As this happens, everything merges into an immense, clear, brilliant light, silent and full of boundless perfection and beauty.

You become one with this light.

You become clear light.

As you practice this exercise in harmonious knowledge, you will discover that your mind and body become flooded with energy, happiness, and serenity. When you unlock the great inner beauty, you wonder which lies at the bedrock of your consciousness. You discover your humanity and the boundless compassion that flows through you. You can then offer this to others.

Compassion is a tree, rejuvenation the fruit that grows on it.

High energy, deep focus, and lasting concentration are the seeds of that fruit.

This tree never dies or withers but is merely overgrown by brambles of the mind.

George was a retired professor of biology whose work was concerned with the very earliest cellular aspects of life. He had traveled the world in search of the meaning of life. Yet, he never felt satisfied. He became very successful, wrote books that sold well, went through three marriages and had four children, and still he wondered what his life was all about.

George had felt tired for most of his life. His mind was razor sharp, but his emotions were blunt and his soul was worn out. He felt separate from people around him and, more important, that he could not trust anyone. So he isolated himself and expected the worst from people and from life, and the worst possible circumstances for himself.

Through Tibetan medicine, he learned that his negative way of viewing the world had become his belief system and that it was only a matter of time before all his worst-case scenarios became worst-case actualities. Bad fortune had plagued George for over two years and he was at a loss to explain it. He moaned that he had done everything in his power to improve his situation, but nothing had changed. Indeed, he had done everything he could think of. But he had not looked within himself. He could not use his inner energies because he didn't know how.

When he discovered how to activate his inner high energy by this meditation, he was first surprised and then shocked at the outcome. For the first time, he discovered that his mind was more than intellect; it was a living, active experience connecting him to boundless energy and a happiness that was not dependent on the world around him.

His run of bad fortune lost its sting, and he realized that his belief in its power had kept him feeling downhearted and unhappy. As his fortune changed, he created positive energy, which made him able to make a better life for himself. He understood that he had more choices in his life, and the business of living became a sacred experience. So George cured himself of the negative emotions and thoughts that were making his life a toxic experience. He does the meditation on a daily basis.

Elizabeth was a singer who lost her voice and didn't know where to find it. One day her voice was normal. She sang without any problems. When she woke up the next day, her voice just wasn't there. She had a concert to do the following evening; all the tickets had been sold.

Without her voice Elizabeth felt as if she were nothing. She felt abandoned by the talent on which she based her identity, career, and reputation. She was plunged into a dark hole from which she felt she had no way out; she felt that no one would understand. She was overcome by such fear that she could hardly move.

Her manager dragged her to see me. The first thing she did after I took her through the meditation exercise was to cry, squeak, and bellow like a pig that has just realized that the farmer has invited it for lunch—and it is the lunch. After this dramatic explosion of sound and emotion, her voice slowly creaked back into life. She did her concert, and now as she tours the world she does this meditation every time before she sings.

Elizabeth learned that her voice fled because she denied her own spirituality. She had to give it a voice. When she *discovered the essential qualities, she felt, in her own words, "connected to the divine."*

Using these techniques allows each of us to connect with the divine in our own ways. Through that connection we find the essence of living. Our minds, bodies, and spirits are refreshed and rejuvenated.

CHAPTER EIGHT

Food and Diet

We live in a society that is extremely anxious about diet. We worry about all manner of things: whether or not to take supplements, eat fats, choose organic produce, and avoid food additives. On and on goes the list, a litany of uncertainty and confusion.

The last seventy years have brought a revolution in how food is grown, processed, and distributed in the West. Much of it is stuffed with compounds ranging from colorings and preservatives to growth hormones and antibiotics. Supermarkets dominate our food-buying habits, and many consumers have become used to paying the lowest possible prices. We have a wide variety of foods to choose from, but what of their quality and health-giving value? Do the foods we choose give us vitality?

Tibetan medicine looks at it like this: Every food on the planet, in either raw or processed form, leaves its effects in the body long after it has left the body. Foods alter, transform, and determine how the body works. Whatever you eat or drink becomes a psychosomatic process. The entire origin and history of the foods and beverages that you have ingested are now part of your consciousness and physical body. So the foods that you eat, how you feel about them, and how you behave when you prepare and eat them directly affect your state of health. The principles of Tibetan medicine can help you to use the nutrients and energies in your foods to make your body and mind happy and cultivate well-being.

In the modern world, particularly in the West, the range now far exceeds the foods available in pre-Communist Tibet. The foods mentioned in this chapter go beyond the confines of traditional Tibetan dietary teaching, but the rules apply in the same way.

Tibetan Dietary Therapy

Tibetan dietary therapy is often the first medical therapy to be used, depending on the personality of the patient, his medical condition, and his circumstances. In a suitable patient, the aim of dietary therapy is to increase vitality through a balanced diet. Modification of diet, if correctly diagnosed, will itself modify unskillful behavior in the patient. Dietary changes can not only prevent internal disease from developing but help to overcome most of the symptoms affecting the ill person.

Equally, food can cause illness. Insufficient, unnecessary, or unsuitable dietary choices will create disease. This comes about through a range of factors, such as not eating enough of the right foods and drinks for the patient's humoral type, under-eating, going on crash diets, or eating too much food continually or in a single sitting.

The Tibetans teach that it is crucial to know when to eat and when not to eat, how much to eat, and also never to overeat. It sounds simple, but many people the world over have no idea of how to implement this concept.

Your body should not be overloaded with excess food. A healthy way of eating is to make sure that your stomach is filled to three-quarters of its capacity. Half of this capacity should be filled by nutritious food, a quarter filled by liquids. This will improve your physical and mental clarity.

Happy Eating

Remember, it's not just what you eat but how you eat it. The focus and care that you give your food returns to you. Healthful foods and fresh juices mindlessly devoured will give less benefit to your body than a lovingly made and consumed hamburger and fries, especially with a large, thick milk shake you have whipped up yourself.

Additionally, your emotional states, habits, and eating patterns can change food to become bad for you. You could end up eating your own anger, unhappiness, fear, and loneliness. Never be angry when you are just about to eat because you will also poison others with your mood. Go somewhere else and be angry, then come back and eat. When you are eating, your mind should be filled with clarity and peace.

Natural Is Best

According to Tibetan dietary wisdom, food takes on the energy of the way in which it is processed or stored. This energy—positive or negative—is then passed on to the consumer. The more naturally the food is processed, the more complete the health benefits it will give.

The eating of food connects all the individuals who made it possible for you to eat. In a perfect situation, the fewer the people in the food chain, from grower to table, the better it is for health and happiness. And that is a big argument for choosing organic, locally grown foods whenever possible.

SEASONAL EATING

The best health comes about by eating in harmony with the seasons. But seasonal eating has largely faded, thanks to supermarkets' being able to supply all foods throughout the year. Even if you don't go the whole way, you can still integrate some seasonal eating to benefit your body, mind, and spirit.

We can all picture the foods we associate with winter, spring, summer, and autumn. Simply choose the vegetables, fruits, nuts, seeds, dairy products, meats, and fish that appeal to you and that are appropriate for each season.

RAW FOODS

Tibetan medicine teaches that raw foods can carry unseen organisms that can poison the body or, if not actually poison it, cause severe changes to the digestive tract and the three humors if eaten regularly. So raw foods, such as salads or uncooked meat or vegetables, are not part of the Tibetan dietary concept, unless particular herbs are used to make them more compatible.

Cooked or partially cooked foods, however, encourage humoral balance and digestive warmth. Refrigeration represses these qualities and confuses the energies of the food, so it's better to let food warm to room temperature if you can, rather than eat it straight from the fridge.

The Seven Bodily Constituents

At the heart of Tibetan dietary therapy are the seven bodily constituents. The theory is very complex, so I have simplified the basic concepts. This will enable you to think about your body and mind in a new way.

The bodily constituents are the active processes in the body that give rise to health or imbalances. They are:

1. *Dangs-ma:* crucial nutrients from ingested food.

2. *Khrag:* blood made from the essential forces of *Dangs-ma*

3. *Sha:* muscle tissues built by the primary qualities of blood.

4. *Tshil:* a particular type of fat tissue involved in the creation of muscles.

5. *Rus:* the many different types of body fats that create bone structure and control bone growth.

6. *rKang:* the types of marrow made from the formative structure of bones.

7. *Khu-ba:* rejuvenating fluids, both reproductive and systemic, created by the pith of bodily marrow.

According to Tibetan medicine, the seven bodily constituents are an alchemic blueprint from which physical, spiritual, and psychological health comes. They are the messengers of health and disease, they control and influence aging, and they are the means to radiant health, good skin, and a balanced mind.

The seven bodily constituents are created by powerful unconscious forces that come from both the brain and the body in a cycle of continual renewal from conception to death. Equally, they hold wisdom within them that is released into the conscious mind and body. So our beings are made up of this constant ever-changing cycle of the seven bodily constituents.

The Tibetan medical system considers the metabolism within the processes of the seven bodily constituents. Each constituent gives a special rebirth to the nutrients as they go through this sevenfold cycle of physical transformation. All of the major organs and body systems are directly connected to this process and refine each stage of the cycle. Each cycle results in by-products and waste products, which are then eliminated.

When a cycle becomes dysfunctional, there is potential for illness. From a Tibetan medical viewpoint, many illnesses can be found in the dysfunctions or malfunctions of the metabolic cycle, because it links brain and body, perceptions and senses to the fragile constructs of the personality.

Digestion, for example, is often a crucial key in this process. Poor nutrition creates poor digestion and poor digestion creates poor nutrition. This has many effects in a person's life on every level, psychological, emotional, intellectual, and physical. It can cause many physical health problems and also damage a person's life force so that he is unable to fulfill them himself.

Tibetan medicine aims to correct long-term problems in the metabolic cycle of a patient's health so that harmony of mind and body become regenerated through the self-correcting functions of the metabolism and the seven bodily constituents. By improving the digestive and nutritional cycle, the body is capable of returning itself to health.

David had suffered from poor digestion for years and had also developed a minor but painful bowel problem. He decided to follow Tibetan dietary wisdom and instead of eating raw food, he heated it gently. He also ate less food.

Not only was he not irritating his digestive system but he was able to absorb more nutrients from his food. His digestive problems improved, his skin, hair, and nails became much more healthy, and he generally had much more vitality.

Each of the seven constituents creates a spiritual, physical, and psychological dimension, and it is these seven multidimensions of the constituents that act as a link with our bodies and minds. The psychological dimension of every constituent is supported by the humors. In this way the constituents influence our senses, emotions, reflexes, and autoimmune systems. As the foundations of metabolism, their effects are so profound that, as they are processed in all the mental and physical systems, they also process and influence one's life.

The constituents link the three humors with your body type and through this interface can help guide you to the types of food that will best suit your physical health, optimum weight, and mental well-being. In the spiritual dimension of each body type, the humors are elevated to support spiritual change. You may find your characteristics in more than one body type, as with the humors, but one will be dominant.

Eating well boosts the seven bodily constituents and supports all of their activities, but a poor diet can destroy the constituents and result in poor emotional and physical health.

Find Your Body Type and Your Psychological and Spiritual Dimensions

Dangs-ma

Crucial nutrients from ingested food. (This refers to both the function and the process of absorbing nutrients.)

Body type: Tall, thin, angular bones, slightly gangly, long limbs, slow-moving, never gains weight regardless of type of food or amount consumed. This body type is influenced by joint conditions. Pale skin with a far-away, wistful look. Camouflages body with loose-fitting clothes.

Spiritual dimension: This most essential physical function is purity and integrity. This refers to the inner knowledge that enables you to act in a virtuous and beneficial manner toward yourself and others. It is here that your humors become balanced and these powerful forces start to support you to live a balanced life.

Psychological dimension: The capacity to behave in a nonviolent manner in thought, speech, and action to all people, communicating honestly, clearly, and non-manipulatively.

Khrag

Blood made from the essential forces of Dangs-ma.

Body type: Medium to tall, with a well-proportioned body with wide shoulders, tapering waist, wide hips, and firm muscles; healthy glowing skin, big eyes, and thick lips. This body type is full of energy and always on the move, with a physical movement that is very fluid and expansive. Although the body is powerful, it is never threatening. Men and women look similar. This body type is influenced by rapid changes in body temperature.

Spiritual dimension: The ability to see into the core of someone's suffering and to identify with compassion, wisdom, and spiritual power so that the person can transform himself, without your perceptive insight becoming emotionally attached.

Psychological dimension: The power to overcome ignorance in all its forms and to transform prejudice in all its guises, while still loving your fellow human beings.

Sha

Muscle tissues built by the primary qualities of blood.

Body type: Small stature, delicate features, quick darting eyes, pointed ears, thin lips with strong cheekbones, long fingers and toes. Well-defined torso and full of stamina. Because this body type is very sensitive to food, eating unsuitable foods affects the bodily constituents and causes mood swings or very intense emotions.

Spiritual dimension: The capacity to be humble and serve those less able than you without regret. To be unselfish through loving and to live for others as well as yourself. To avoid being addicted to the charisma that other people attach to you.

Psychological dimension: The determination to go on through hardship as you build yourself or others a new life or consciousness. The ability to love and be loved but not to be owned through loving. It's important not to be overcome by the force of obstructions, but know that they pass by like rain clouds on a summer afternoon.

Tshil

A particular type of fat tissue used in the creation of muscles.

Body type: Tall, slightly overweight, muscular, dominant body, able to influence others through physical presence. Big hands, prominent knuckles and joints, big thrusting chin, big teeth—everything seems large about this body type. Red in face or slightly flushed. Controlled by sexual desires, this body type may also fight with the forces of addiction.

Spiritual dimension: The potential to understand that you cannot own spiritual insight, enlightenment, wisdom, power, or love. You cannot own ownership. All these things you can only pass on.

Psychological dimension: Living well, living your dream, is the act of total responsibility. This dimension drives this body type to try to live their dreams.

Rus

The nature of bone manufacture from particular body fats.

Body type: Of medium height or small, full of physically generated charisma and immense power, this body type is rounded, curvy, and smooth, sometimes prone to excess body fluids or fats. Adaptable to its immediate environment and able to eat whatever is available without getting ill. This body type is a gauge of the individual's mood, changing as quickly as a barometer.

Spiritual dimension: The desire runs through you to build a spiritual structure that brings people together and yet helps them to know their individuality. Sacred structures of all kinds are the bones upon which spirituality rests, though only for a short time. A bone grows if well fed, so study the nature of bone growth to know yourself.

Psychological dimension: Remember that because people do not know who they are, they cannot know who you are. Every person is worthy of attention and is due respect.

rKang

The types of marrow made from the formative structures of bones.

Body type: This body type is compact, rigid, and seemingly immovable; mentally has a tendency to be self-obsessed. Dense muscle and body, of any height. The body seems stiff but is actually and naturally highly flexible; its dynamic energy is physically but quietly expressed.

Spiritual dimension: In the marrow lies the truth, the history, the moment, and the future of how things were, are, and shall be. How do you extract the marrow of your soul to know how it is made? Give up ego, pretense, and knowledge, or just study the way your body is? Both, perhaps. Knowing how things are means you can change them.

Psychological dimension: Everything is in the marrow; do you really want to extract it? You don't need to force the way to truth. It is inside you right now.

Khu–ba

Rejuvenating fluids, both reproductive and systemic, created by the pith of bodily marrow.

> *Body type:* This body type looks like a mixture of the others, with slightly flushed skin indicating a strong vitality. This vitality drives both an intense mind and an active body type with speedy reflexes. This body type cannot stand still: everything moves quickly.
>
> *Spiritual dimension:* As your body renews, so does consciousness. As your body dies, so does illusion about consciousness. All things within you are rejuvenated; all things come from that which is the first to die.
>
> *Psychological dimension:* Change is war as far as your mind is concerned. Your everyday mind yells with terror when rejuvenation comes near, for fear that it will not know itself anymore. The imagination of the past holds it back; death without change is preferable to everlasting conscious life. This is what your habitual mind believes. But it can transform itself and know that in this dimension rejuvenation gives birth to consciousness.

Now let us look further into the way in which Tibetan medicine views diet.

The Six Tastes

As we now know from the concept of the seven bodily constituents, when food enters the metabolic system, it goes through a cycle of seven stages, to produce the life and vitality that is essential for this material incarnation.

The crux of the Tibetan theory of food and diet is the concept of six tastes, which condition and influence the seven constituents and in turn the three humors (see below) and the five elements (see chapters 6 and 7).

As I said earlier, all foods have histories and energies that affect many people, particularly processed and other mass-produced foods. They pass on these effects through the six tastes: sweet, sour, salty, bitter, sharp, and astringent. According to Tibetan medicine, these tastes are found in eight groups of foods: grains, beverages, meats, oils and fats, cooked and preserved food, vegetables, fruits, and spices.

The six tastes are closely connected with the digestive cycle. For instance, too much sweetness sedates the digestive cycle, whereas too much sour shocks and diminishes its effectiveness. If you eat too much of a salty taste, your digested food becomes stuck in your gut and poisons you. An excess of bitter, sharp, or astringent taste makes food ferment in your digestive tract, which decreases your vitality and emotional balance.

How to Use the Knowledge of the Six Tastes

The six tastes play an important part in how each of the three humors (Wind, Bile, and Phlegm) influence your body from conception through life and death. As we go through life, the three humors, and your dominant humor, influence how your body changes. Your dominant humor and most dominant taste(s) will indicate what foods are best for you. Tibetan medicine teaches us that although there is no one healthy diet for everyone, there are correct foods for creating health according to the individual's dominant tastes and humors.

The six tastes regulate and shape how your body feels, functions, and looks by influencing metabolism and overall health. Along with each taste in the following pages is an explanation of how Tibetan medicine regards its influence on our bodies, personalities, and lives. As you read this next section, explore which taste or tastes are dominant in your life through the foods you choose to eat. Then you can discover which foods and tastes are good for you when you are ill or under pressure. You will be able to see the way in which the tastes influence your dominant humor and thus your general state of health.

You will notice that several foods—chocolate, citrus fruits, oysters, and spiced meats, for example—occur in more than one group. This is because they contain multiple ingredients that affect people in different ways.

Chocolate was not, of course, known to the Tibetans, but it can be classified according to Tibetan dietary law. Curiously, chocolate and coffee are the only substances that contain all tastes, elements, and humors and so adapt themselves to everyone. Because they are so adaptable, they can alter the mind and body. If taken regularly, they eventually become a poison to which we can become addicted. Rather than cut them out completely, Tibetan medicine suggests using chocolate and coffee in small doses as a medicine to sedate and calm.

THE SIX TASTES AND THEIR PROPERTIES

Sweet (Mngar-ba)

Foods: honey, brown sugar, molasses, chocolate, milk, ice cream, most raw meats, baked foods, bread, rice, barley, lentils, fish, all grains and pulses, fruits (except apricots), tomatoes, avocados, root vegetables including potatoes and carrots, celery, and processed foods.

WHAT SWEET TASTE DOES

This taste influences and controls the rate at which your body converts food to energy. Depending on the humoral influence, your body type will affect whether this is fast, slow, or a combination of the two. This taste makes the body crave either salty things or sweets. Low proteins, low fats, high carbohydrates such as milk, fish, rice, celery, or anything listed under the sweet section, above, are best when the body craves a sweet taste.

Healthy Use

In moderation, sweet foods are nutritious and happy within the body, improving the seven constituents of the body and encouraging them to grow. Sweet foods increase body weight and so are important for the old and young and feeble. Medium-sweet foods, such as milk, rice, and celery, ease sore throats, suppress coughs, and activate wound healing. The medium-sweet quality is an antitoxin; it balances and improves the five senses and balances the Wind and Phlegm humors.

Excess Use: Beware!

If there is an excess of the sweet taste in the diet, it will promote the growth of unhealthy fat and body fluids, diminish body heat and vitality, energize the Bile humor, and contribute to a wide number of lymphatic, glandular, and metabolic disorders, which in turn affect organ function.

Sour

Foods: milk products, chocolate, ice cream, cheeses, lemon and other citrus fruits, hot spices, alcohol, pickled food, vinegars, fish, apricots (based on their effects on digestion), pineapples, passion fruit, mangoes, and berries.

What Sour Taste Does

This taste regulates the metabolism and influences the autonomic nervous system, which regulates cardiac muscle and glands.

HEALTHY USE

In moderation, sour foods can help to develop and maintain body heat and appetite and regulate thirst. This taste also influences the way the body and brain talk to each other and directs the metabolic functions. Sour foods can regulate diarrhea and an unhealthy stomach and influence digestion. Sour augments the touch sense and can also activate the sluggish Wind humor, improving its movement.

EXCESS USE: BEWARE!

In excess, sour foods awaken the Bile humor and influence the Phlegm humor, encouraging physical and mental lethargy. Sour can overstimulate thirst, causing fever and delirium. Nausea and aching limbs are also linked to too much sour taste in the body. Overuse can seriously weaken immune, lymphatic, and metabolic functions of the body and open up the body to infections and serious organ and system dysfunction.

Salty

Foods: salt, chocolate, burned or barbecued foods, fish, cheese, edible seaweed and similar freshwater plants, breakfast cereals, bacon and bacon products, and snack foods.

WHAT SALTY TASTE DOES

This taste influences the anabolic and catabolic functions of the body, which, according to Tibetan medicine, control how your body makes energy. If you are Wind humor dominant, you will have poor sleep if this taste is out of balance; if you are Bile dominant, you will be agitated, and if you are Phlegm dominant you will suffer from constipation or diarrhea. Eat dark green plants to help this balance.

Healthy Use

Many physical obstructions, such as constipation, water reten-
tion, and sore joints, are removed by this taste; it increases the
healthy sweat function of the body, activates appetite, and
maintains body heat.

Excess Use: Beware!

Too much salty food can encourage a wide range of skin
problems connected with the lymphatic system and kidneys,
including flaking, peeling, or thinning skin, and hair loss. In
excess, it encourages premature aging, decreases body weight
through fluid loss, and increases thirst through poor assimi-
lation of fluids. Excess salty taste energizes the Phlegm
humor.

Bitter

Foods: concentrated and preserved foods, chocolate, alcohol,
coffee, Indian black tea (not Chinese or Sri Lankan), lettuce,
watercress, asparagus, broccoli, rocket and similar greens,
and olives.

What Bitter Taste Does

This taste, more than any other, will influence the effectiveness
of your endocrine (hormonal) system, which in turn influences
your body shape and your dominant humor. This taste directs
the body type to be sculptured by the humoral influence.

Healthy Use

In moderation, this taste will improve the appetite, stimulate
memory, stop thirst, limit infections, act as an antibacterial and
antitoxic agent, and stop fainting spells. It will curb excess fat,
grease, bodily fluids, urine, and all forms of excrement, and
also stop the Bile humor from becoming imbalanced.

EXCESS USE: BEWARE!

Too much bitter taste will weaken the body, according to the seven bodily constituents of Tibetan medicine.

Sharp

Foods: pickled foods, alcohol, dry foods, chocolate, snack foods, chilies, garlic, onions, chives, radishes, ginger, leeks, cinnamon, nutmeg, all peppers, and culinary dried herbs.

WHAT SHARP TASTE DOES

This taste will either strengthen or weaken the function of the body's immune system and inflammatory responses.

HEALTHY USE

This taste improves heat to the stomach and gastrointestinal tract and so aids in digestion, increases appetite, and cleans out blocked tubes in the body; the sharp quality helps in healing most throat problems and clears decaying tissue.

EXCESS USE: BEWARE!

In excess, this taste reduces the manufacture of reproductive fluids in men and women, debilitates the body, and increases shivering and fainting. It can decrease mobility in the waist and upper torso. Too much sharp-tasting food can also reduce the vitality in blood and other body fluids and tissue.

Astringent

Foods: red meat, organ meat, sausages, burned food, bacon and other smoked meats, pâté, caviar, seafood, water biscuits, potato chips, chocolate, alcohol, milk products, toast, peanut butter, nuts, seaweed, zucchini, chicory, Brussels sprouts, spring onions, cabbage, pineapple, grapefruit, turmeric, saffron, and gourds.

WHAT ASTRINGENT TASTE DOES

This taste influences the circulatory functions of all the body's systems and its osmotic pressure, the quality of blood, and the amount of useful fluids in the body.

HEALTHY USE

In moderation, this taste helps wound-healing in joints and organs, depression, and low energy. It heals bad complexions and adult acne, gives shine and radiance to the complexion, and helps the skin stay young.

EXCESS USE: BEWARE!

In excess, astringent foods increase any sensation of bloating of the intestines and stomach and contribute to puffiness of the abdomen. This taste restricts bodily channels and tubes, encourages weak stomachs and constipation, and quickly debilitates the body. The astringent quality can stimulate over-production of mucus and lymph, causing flatulence and excess gas of the upper digestive tract, angina, and unstable heartbeat. In general, too much astringent food contributes to coronary disorders and rapid, unsafe, and irregular heart function. It may also lead to foggy thinking.

HEALING STRESS BY CHOOSING THE RIGHT TASTE AT THE RIGHT TIME

Major life changes carry with them stress, which can lead to different forms of poor health, such as weight gain and loss, which we look at in the following pages. Eating the right food at these times can lessen the hurt and shock and increase the opportunities for balance and healing. Tibetan medicine believes that if you crave a certain taste during a time of stress, it is a symbolic guide to something you should do or should be, in order to enhance or to help solve the situation.

For example, if you crave something sweet-tasting in a crisis, it may be that a "sweet" action would soften the intensity and soothe the crisis. You can apply the same thinking to the other tastes. So, just as sweet would create peace and conciliation, sour would wake up protagonists and make them see sense. Salty would help them see the facts, bitter would reveal if there was any bitterness fueling dissent, sharp would shock the complacent, and astringent would reveal the truth in people's hearts.

BALANCING IMBALANCES

If you feel unbalanced, examine how you feel in the context of the six tastes. Do you feel sweet, sour, salty, bitter, sharp, or astringent? Choose what seems the most apt in describing your state of mind, then eat the opposite:

- If you desire the sweet taste, eat astringent.
- If you desire the sour taste, eat sharp.
- If you desire the salty taste, eat bitter.
- If you desire the bitter taste, eat sweet.
- If you desire the sharp taste, eat salty.
- If you desire the astringent taste, eat sharp.

The reverse of this list is also true. This will help to bring balance.

Using the tastes symbolically in this way can act as a powerful channel to your inner knowledge, bringing understanding and insight about situations.

Stress-related Weight Loss and Gain

Stress is as old as humankind and exists in some way in every culture. The ancient Tibetans developed a huge range of stress-busting techniques. One of the most effective is to help heal yourself with food. Tibetan medicine says that the more anxious we are, the more our humors are out of balance. Then one or more of the six tastes will grow in dominance and damage the seven bodily constituents, causing weight problems.

According to Tibetan medicine, two things tend to happen when you get stressed: You either lose or put on a lot of weight. This happens if you eat the wrong foods, which can devitalize the brain and nervous system so that they work poorly. If, for instance, the sweet taste becomes dominant, the body stores more nutrients and these turn into fat. If the sweet taste actually becomes in control of the other tastes, excess fat is deposited deep in the abdomen.

If people put on a lot of weight very quickly because of stress, their major glandular systems are sick. According to Tibetan medicine, they need professional help.

Eating the right food when you're stressed, however, can dissolve tension, increase energy, balance mood swings, and help sleep problems. To counter stress-related weight gain or loss, eat any of the astringent, sharp, and sour foods listed above, in any combination, over a ten-day period.

Healing the Stresses of Life with Food for Your Humoral Type

In chapter 6 you found your dominant humoral type. To help optimize your health and prevent illness, eat the foods in your category, below, as the foundation of your daily diet.

WIND FOODS (YELLOW, ORANGE, WHITE)

Apricots, pineapples, papayas, mangoes, apples, bananas, citrus fruits, plantains, sweet corn, maize, honey, chicken, quail, duck, goose, egg yolks, fish eggs (but not caviar), butter, buttermilk, and ghee.

BILE FOODS (PINK, RED, DARK RED)

Cooked prawns, caviar, pink- or red-fleshed fish, cooked lamb, red onions, red cabbage, tomatoes, red peppers, cherries, red grapes, watermelon, red plums, pink grapefruit, small amounts of red wine, and any other pink, red, or dark red foods, including red berries.

PHLEGM FOODS (BLUE, PURPLE, DARK BROWN)

Blackberries, boysenberries, blueberries, aubergines, dates, figs, molasses, seeds, nuts, pure chocolate (70 percent cocoa or over), rye, rye bread(sour dough), organ meats including livers, hearts, offal, lamb kidneys and brains, and any other foods of this color.

IMMEDIATE FOOD MEDICINES

Tibetan medicine encourages us to eat foods that regulate our cycles of eating. The foods below act as immediate "medicines" to balance and increase vitality. Eat them regularly as part of your diet at the times recommended.

Dairy products: Best eaten in the early morning for breakfast and at dinner in the evening. Yogurts, cheese, and milk from sheep, cows, goats, and oxen.

Meat, poultry, fish, game: Best eaten in the morning for breakfast or early lunch, then in the early evening for supper. For sick people or growing children, red meat or venison or game with a little fat is essential to make the brain function and so create a healthy mind and body; fat on meat fights infections when it is cooked properly. The leanest meat possible is best for healthy adults. According to Tibetan medicine, it is good to eat meat with fruit, cooked or uncooked, but not with a lot of root vegetables.

Oily fish: Fish such as salmon, sea trout, tuna, sardines, pilchards, and herring.

Fruit: Eat small amounts throughout the day. Fruit brings peace to the body and mind and, in moderation, is good for stimulating the body to break down excess fat. However, it should not be used as a main food supply (e.g., as in fruitarianism) because it can overstimulate the sweet taste, sedating the digestive tract and making the consumer vacant and directionless.

Vegetables: Eat regularly at breakfast, lunch, and dinner. Root vegetables cooked in a low-temperature oven for a long time are good for general health. All vegetables are best made into soup, or cooked lightly, rather than raw.

Pulses and beans: Eat on their own or mixed with meat; do not mix with other vegetables, as this creates imbalances in the six tastes and seven bodily constituents.

Grains: Rice, oats, barley, millet, corn, buckwheat, quinoa, and wheat heal the body and mind rapidly, encouraging balance. Eat on their own or with meat or fish; do not mix with pulses or beans. Do not mix with dairy products, as in breakfast cereals and milk. Long-term eating of milk mixed with grains creates a dominant sweet taste in the body, leading to stress, low energy, and poor concentration, due to poor bodily function. According to Tibetan medicine, the practice of mixing additives with wheat in breakfast cereals, pastries, snack bars, and other prepared foods that creates a sweet taste is the cause of the wheat allergies that affect so many people nowadays. Grains relax the nervous system, increase energy, direct the seven bodily nutrients to the brain, and encourage balanced behavior and refreshing sleep.

Food is a vehicle to self-knowledge and healing. Understanding how the seven bodily constituents, the six tastes, and the three humors connect will empower you to make better choices in food, diet, and health.

CHAPTER NINE

DIY Remedies and Self-help Techniques

Many Tibetan healing techniques evolved to help people solve minor problems when they were many days' journey from a physician. So there is a rich store of traditional remedies for treating yourself and your family. Here are some simple ways in which you can use herbs, spices, massage, and hydrotherapy, as well as color and sound.

Herbal Medicines

All living things are sacred, including the medicinal plants of the world. As well as adding flavor to our foods, herbs and spices are medicines for the mind and body. The wisdom of ancient systems, such as Tibetan medicine, teaches us that we have much to learn by developing an empathic and intuitive connection with plants.

Like animals, all plants teach us about our place in the world. Medicinal plants can allow us to access information about ourselves as well as balance our bodies. Using such herbs can help us to reflect on our lives, our health, and our states of happiness and unhappiness.

The survival of mankind over the millennia depended on using plants as medicine. The pharmaceutical industry was originally based on phytochemistry, and a significant proportion of mainstream drugs today are still made directly from plant sources. Rather than buy them over the counter, you can follow the lead of our ancestors—as many people in the world still do—and use herbs and other medicinal plants to treat simple ills.

Tibetan herbal medicine is a vast and complex store of knowledge, but there are safe remedies you can make at home, using easily found herbs and spices. The purpose of these decoctions and pills is not to bury the condition but rather to encourage the body and mind to heal. Some patients may feel worse before getting better, but this is nothing to worry about. This response is due to the medicine working to create the right balance in the body and to harmonize body and mind.

Please remember that these remedies are for minor health problems that are normally short-lived. If problems do not improve or seem to worsen, consult your doctor or other health professional immediately.

STORE CUPBOARD

There are a number of dried herbs and spices that you should keep in your store cupboard to use for a range of common problems: basil (dried but not powdered), cardamom pods (black and green), cloves (whole), chili powder, cinnamon powder, coriander (dried leaf or powder), cumin powder, garlic powder, ginger powder, juniper berries, licorice sticks, mustard powder, peppercorns (or ground pepper), saffron strands, sage powder, turmeric powder, and raw organic honey.

These can be made into decoctions to fight the conditions below.

How to Make a Decoction

Bring one pint (570 ml) of fresh filtered water to a boil over low heat. Cover as it starts to boil and turn off the heat. Cool until completely cold to remove any possible germs and negative energy. Heat the water to a boil again, adding the herbs as below. Cool, strain, and use as needed. Store in a clean container in a dark cupboard or in the refrigerator. The decoction will stay fresh and safe to use for a maximum of three days, depending on the weather.

AILMENTS AND THEIR TREATMENTS

Common Cold

To the boiling water, add one level teaspoon of turmeric, five strands of saffron, one stick of licorice, one teaspoon of sage, one teaspoon of cumin, and three cloves. Cover and simmer for fifteen minutes, then turn off the heat, let it stand until cold, and strain.

Dosage:

- Children over ten years old and adults, two teaspoons of the decoction every two hours until symptoms improve.

- Children from five years to ten years, one teaspoon of the decoction in one tablespoon cool water, three times daily after meals plus a last cup before bed.

- Very old or frail people and babies from one year old to five years, one teaspoon of the decoction in one tablespoon of warm milk, three times a day after meals.

Warning: Do not give to infants under one year old; it is too strong and will make them ill.

Minor Chest Infections

Put five cardamom pods into boiling water as above, sprinkle a quarter of a teaspoon of chili powder into the water, and add three juniper berries, half a teaspoon of garlic powder, five strands of saffron, three sticks of licorice, and one teaspoon of cinnamon. Simmer for twenty minutes, cool, then strain.

Dosage:

- Adults, three teaspoons of the decoction, taken every hour.

- Children from five to ten years, one teaspoon of the decoction, in one teaspoon of cool water, before each meal or snack.

- Children from 10 to 18, two tablespoons of the decoction in two tablespoons of warm water, every two hours.

- Elderly adults, one tablespoon of the decoction in one tablespoon of warm water, every four hours.

Warning: This remedy is not suitable for children under age five.

Poor Sleep

To the boiling water, as above, add three sticks of licorice, seven saffron strands, one tablespoon of dark brown organic honey, and half a teaspoon of cinnamon, then simmer for 15 minutes. Let cool until lukewarm and strain.

Dosage:
- Drink one cup on the hour for three hours before you go to bed.

Sores

To the boiling water, add three teaspoons each of basil, sage, ginger, turmeric, garlic, and pepper (white or black). Simmer for 20 minutes, then strain.

How to use:
- With a clean cloth, apply the fluid to the affected areas five times daily. Alternatively, soak a cloth in the mixture and place it on the sore for one hour; apply a fresh damp cloth four times a day.

Dosage:
- For adults and children over ten, drink four teaspoons of the decoction in two tablespoons warm water, four times daily with meals.

Warning: Do not drink on an empty stomach.

Cuts and Abrasions

To the boiling water, add 4 teaspoons of turmeric, 2 teaspoons of mustard, and 2 teaspoons of ginger. Simmer for 20 minutes on low heat. Cool and strain. This mild disinfectant is excellent for killing infections from minor cuts and abrasions. Apply with clean cloth as needed.

Warning: Do not drink.

Constant Fatigue

If you lack vitality and feel tired all the time, the following decoction may help. Into the boiling water, put four sticks of licorice, three teaspoons of coriander, four cardamom pods, ten saffron strands, and a pinch of grated nutmeg. Simmer for 25 minutes, cool, and strain.

Dosage:
- One tablespoon every four hours for three days; then drink four cups a day for ten days.

STORE CUPBOARD

The following ingredients should be powdered or ground: basil, cardamom (black and green), chili, cinnamon, cloves, coriander, cumin, garlic, ginger, juniper berries, licorice sticks, mustard, pepper (black and white), saffron, sage, turmeric, plus raw organic honey, black molasses, and corn, barley, or rice flour.

These can be made into tablets in order to treat a range of common health problems.

How to Make Simple Tablets

You can mix herbs with rice or barley flour, honey, and black molasses to make simple pills. The base is two tablespoons of black molasses and honey (about one tablespoon each) mixed with one tablespoon of barley or rice flour.

Add one teaspoon of each herb in the following recipes, except saffron. Up to twenty strands of saffron should be added, either cut or broken into small pieces, but not chopped.

Roll the mixture into pea-sized balls and dust with a little more of the flour. Store on a flat tray until dry. You can either leave them in the sunlight or speed the process by putting them in the oven on the lowest possible heat for up to ten minutes, then let them dry in the air. Once hard, each tablet will last up to two years.

The tablets can be swallowed with a little water.

Ailments and Their Treatments

Sore Throats

Blend together one teaspoon each of cloves, black pepper, turmeric, and coriander, then mix into the base.

Dosage:
- Take one pill four times a day, just before eating and before bed, with a little water.

Poor Digestion and Flatulence

Mix together one teaspoon each of sage, cumin, coriander, and cinnamon, and five saffron strands. Blend with the base.

Dosage:
- Take one pill every three hours.

Herbal Fire

Both Buddhist and Bön medicine use herbs spiritually and ritualistically. When my teacher used herbs for rituals he would have a fire burning for a long time. When it had burned down, he would sprinkle on the herbs and incant mantras to invoke the deities and spirits of the elements or to heal people or situations from a distance.

You can simply sprinkle a little of any of the herbs on charcoal, on a live fire, or carefully on a candle flame. Here are some simple suggestions:

Turmeric: For low moods, negative environments, and blocked sinuses. If you feel depressed and don't know why, or you feel that your environment is full of negative thoughts, sprinkle a little turmeric on a flame, as above. The acrid smell clears confusion. Inhaling the aroma clears the sinuses.

Ginger: For shock, conflict, and sore throats. Burn some powdered ginger as above to clear shock and emotional pain. The bittersweet fragrance will also help to unite people who are separated by arguments and to heal broken trust. Ginger drives out divisive energy. Inhaling its smoke is good for sore throats.

Saffron: For purifying the environment and strengthening weak eyes and lungs. Burn ten strands of saffron as above or simply ignite a little pile of strands with a match, to create an influx of higher spiritual energy that will purify the environment. The dark, pervasive smell of burning saffron brings love and breaks down obstructions and fear. Inhaling its smoke is good for weak eyes and weak lungs.

Garlic: For violent thoughts, unwelcome people, and germs. The smoke of burned garlic drives away violent thoughts and action and cleanses the environment of germs and the imprints of undesirable people. Inhaling its sweet smell calms nervous people and reduces psychological pain.

Cinnamon: Burning this spice brings harmony and creativity, encourages happiness, and brings clarity of mind and energy.

Nutmeg: Burning nutmeg stimulates shifts in perception about complex problems. It attracts money to the place where it is burned, but that also brings the responsibility of wealth, so you must be prepared to work for and with that money. Inhaling nutmeg may improve skin infections.

Black and/or white pepper: Burning either type of pepper encourages learning and concentration. Its acrid, pungent smell removes bad odors from the environment. Inhaling the aroma can help to heal mouth ulcers.

Basil and sage: When burned, these herbs relieve stress and change discord into joviality. They encourage memories from the past to resurface, engendering sentimental thoughts. If inhaled they can act as an aphrodisiac, stimulating powerful displays of sexual passion. The aroma can also influence people toward acts of piety and kindness. These herbs can enable you to influence other people in the immediate environment.

Ground or whole juniper berries: Juniper has many sacred uses in Tibetan spiritual beliefs; in Buddhist and Bön teachings, this herb is used to invoke deities, purify buildings, and create a sacred environment. The sweet dry smell of the berries can induce a state of concentration that aids meditation, prayer, or any form of worship.

DIY Massage and Other Self-help Techniques

In modern times, massage has been relegated to a lesser role in Tibetan medicine, but it is still regarded highly by many Tibetans. It can be used for all ages, from infancy to old age. Massage has the power to ameliorate all manner of physical conditions, both acute and chronic, as well as stress-related problems and severe psychological or psychiatric conditions. It is also used to prevent illness and for general well-being.

There are many different massage techniques in Tibetan medicine, and an experienced practitioner will use different forms as part of treatment, but let us focus on what you can do for yourself and for your family and friends. It's simple to do and completely free.

WHOLE BODY MASSAGE FOR VITALITY AND WELL-BEING

You don't need to use oil but, if you do, it's best to use an unscented massage oil. Using the palm of your hand, massage with counterclockwise circular movements away from the heart.

Start with your torso, then go on to your neck, arms, wrists, hands, and fingers. Use your right hand to massage the left side of your body and limbs, and vice versa (if you are massaging another person, use the hand that feels most comfortable). Rub around the edges of each finger and the fingertips with the opposite palm. Next, move to your inner and outer thighs, middle to lower back (starting wherever you can reach), then your buttocks, legs, heels, ankles, feet, and toes.

Do this as vigorously as you can for ten minutes, twice daily, for ten days, when you wake up and just before you go to sleep. It will improve circulation and body tone, help to balance the three humors, aid digestion, calm stress, and, in general, enhance your body's ability to work and rest.

At the end of ten days, take a two-day break so that your body can absorb all of the benefits of the massage, then repeat the process.

This massage is safe for everyone, so make it a regular health habit for you and your family or friends. For old people and babies, or anyone else in fragile physical health, massage carefully and gently. When you are massaging other people, keep a slow rhythmic movement and ask them about the pressure they prefer. Try to feel the shapes and contours of their bodies.

Tibetan Acupressure for Minor Complaints

The Tibetan form of acupressure is safe, simple, and helps to boost well-being and relieve minor problems. This traditional self-healing technique was developed thousands of years ago by the homemakers and farmers of Tibet. They used it as an effective treatment when they or their family or neighbors were ill or in pain and a physician was not on hand. Later, the system was adopted and refined by physicians.

As with all acupressure systems, the points are on channels (or meridians) that relate to physiological and energetic structures of the mind and body. The Tibetan system is based on the flow of the three humors, elemental energies, and pulse functions.

How to Give Yourself Acupressure

Use your index finger or your thumb, or both together, pressing down firmly on the point as you count to 100 slowly. Release for the count of 10, then repeat five times.

Conditions treated: Nausea, diarrhea, stomach pain and gas caused by overeating, bad food, or mild poisoning.

Acupressure point: Center of each palm and on each fingertip.

Conditions treated: Travel sickness, headaches caused by the common cold.

Acupressure point: Middle of each wrist, upper and lower, and each earlobe, front and back.

Condition treated: Mild joint pain.

Acupressure point: Middle of each inner elbow.

Conditions treated: Poor vitality, muscle pain, stress-related conditions.

Acupressure point: Either side of the chest above the breastbone.

Conditions treated: Blocked sinuses, insomnia, sleeplessness.

Acupressure point: Midpoint between your eyebrows.

Conditions treated: Overwhelming fatigue, anxiety, headache, upper neck pain.

Acupressure point: Middle of your forehead, just below your hairline.

Conditions treated: Stiff neck, frozen shoulder, stiff shoulders and arms.

Acupressure point: Base of your neck where it meets your spine.

Conditions treated: Muscular pain in the spine, general stiffness.

Acupressure point: Either side of the spine in the middle of your back.

Condition treated: Back pain.

Acupressure point: Middle of each buttock.

Condition treated: Sore or stiff legs.

Acupressure point: Middle of the folds behind each knee.

Conditions treated: Toothache, backache, constipation.

Acupressure point: Middle of each instep.

Condition treated: General debilitation.

Acupressure point: Tip of each big toe.

Conditions treated: Overindulgence, chronic illness, joint injury, repetitive injury (such as repetitive strain injury or RSI), continual hurt to the back.

Acupressure point: Middle of each sole, four times a day.

Hydrotherapy

Hydrotherapy was and is still used in Tibetan medicine to restore vitality to illnesses caused by the three humors, Wind, Bile, and Phlegm. Typically, these might be stress or addictions of any kind that result from Wind imbalance, joint problems, digestive disorders, or skin conditions related to Bile problems, or infections leading from a Phlegm disorder. In ancient times, a physician would sometimes instruct a patient to stand under a powerful waterfall, to be sponged in hot or cold water, or to sit in a Tibetan sauna. Today, you can use Tibetan hydrotherapy techniques if you have access to a sauna and a powerful shower.

Hydrotherapy guidelines:

- Do not use a sauna after you have drunk alcohol (even a small amount) or eaten food. Always drink 1.75 pints (1 litre) of pure water before doing these hydrotherapy treatments and 3.5 pints (2 litres) in the two hours following your sauna.

- Always rest for at least fifteen minutes after doing any of these hydrotherapy treatments.

Safe and Simple Detoxes Using a Shower or Sauna

For joint problems, skin conditions, and general fatigue:

- Stand under a warm shower for ten minutes.
- Without drying yourself, go straight into the sauna for five minutes.
- Repeat this cycle five times.
- Thoroughly towel yourself dry; do not worry if you sweat a little.

For stress and the common cold, to prevent flu and bronchitis, to ease the effects of rheumatism and arthritis in the early stages, and to aid recovery from long-term illness:

- Take a hot shower, as hot you can stand it, for exactly two minutes.
- Go straight into the sauna for two minutes.

- Take a very cold shower, as cold as you can, for two minutes.

- Go into the sauna for exactly five minutes.

- Take a warm shower for five minutes.

- Go back into the sauna for a minimum of three minutes, up to ten minutes if you can.

- Towel yourself dry thoroughly.

For hangovers but *not* if you are still very drunk in the morning:

- If you feel ill or have a mild hangover, drink two glasses of warm water mixed with lemon juice or strong ginger tea.

- Shower in very warm water for ten minutes.

- Go straight into the sauna for five minutes.

- Take a lukewarm shower for ten minutes.

- Go back into the sauna for five minutes.

- Take a hot shower for one minute.

- Towel yourself dry thoroughly and vigorously.

- Drink lots of water, then rub the soles and balls of your feet very hard, ten times on each foot.

For the effects of anxiety, panic, stress, and fatigue brought on by shock, work, or any other life experience:

- Undress and towel yourself all over your body as hard as you can with a clean rough towel. Don't leave out any part of your body, including the top of your head, behind your ears, ankles, feet and toes, hands and fingers, lips and nose.

- Take some fresh basil or sage leaves into a hot shower.

- Stroke the herbs all over your body as you shower for one minute. The water must be as hot as you can handle.

- Go straight into the sauna with your basil or sage leaves, tear them up, and rub them all over your body. Take what is left and put them in a little pile near you.

- Sit quietly in the sauna for eight to fifteen minutes, inhaling the aroma of the herbs.

- Shower in warm water for five minutes.

- Towel yourself dry vigorously.

Tibetan Color Healing, Moon Power, and the Seasons

According to Tibetan wisdom, every season has a color. Although the Tibetan calendar and season organization are different from ours, the wisdom of the seasons translates very well, so we can use the colors to balance our humors and create good fortune in our careers, personal lives, and spiritual endeavors.

Winter: December to Early February

Winter is the season of insight and the maturing of wisdom. It is the time for reflection and balance. This is the time to consider your actions and plan for the future based on your past experiences. It is also the time to purify yourself.

The winter full moon is white, so, each month, put white flowers, fabric, or objects in your home or workplace. Tune in to the full moon by reflecting on it and the white objects, thinking how they may purify your mind and body and the environment around you.

At the end of the full moon cycle, place a white flower or a little piece of white cloth into running water; this removes your impurities and creates positive energy.

Spring: Mid-February to End of April

Spring is the cycle of happiness and discovery. All things can be healed in this season.

The color for spring is red. On the day of each new moon in springtime, fill your house or workplace with red objects. Wear red if you wish. Focus on the new moon, on its symbolic red color, and its capacity to bring you all the vitality of spring, heal you, cleanse your mind and body, and lead you to happiness.

To strengthen the effect, bury one of the red objects you used in this exercise in your garden or in a pot of soil; this will bring you the power of spring throughout the year.

Summer: May to October

The nature of summer is one of expansion, realization, and conscious awareness of who you are and what you can be. It is the reminder that all things come to a fruitful apex before they fade away to be born again. Summer is the season of birth and death, of renewal and reconstruction and resurrection—a reminder that all energy reincarnates through differing forms.

Gold is the color for summer. In the first few weeks of summer, fill your house and place of work with golden objects, reflecting the color of the summer moons. On each waxing moon, tune in to the unfolding of prosperity and feel at one with yourself, the world, and the universe. The moon will bring you contentment, insight about the way you live, and protection of your household and loved ones. Just before the end of summer, in the last few days of October, place one of the gold-colored objects into a fire and it will release the energy of abundance and connection with nature.

Autumn: End of October to Start of December

Autumn is very dark green in color. On each waning moon, fill your home and workplace with dark green objects and wear something of that color.

The waning moons can give you a connection to the power of autumn. Tune in to November's waning moon and draw its powerful energy to you so that your problems, obstructions, and difficulties are washed away.

On the last waning moon of this season (you can check this in a lunar calendar; many diaries and astrology columns also include this information), take a piece of green fabric or some green seeds and cast them into the autumnal winds so that they are scattered far and wide. As you do so, infuse these objects with all the energy that you have created throughout this autumn lunar ritual. In this way, you are spreading the power and blessing.

Healing with Sound and Vibration

Sound is vibration. Nature is vibration. Billions of vibrations give you shape and form. Tibetan medicine has used this knowledge since ancient times. However, the formal version of sound and vibrational healing is a very profound and ancient skill that only a true master should carry out. Rather than try expert techniques such as overtone chanting, you can simply tune in to the sounds of nature that are all around you, all the time.

Here is a simple and safe method for tuning in to sounds

and subtle vibrations in order to heal and harmonize yourself. Sit comfortably in a chair, with your back supported and your feet flat on the floor. Close your eyes. Raise your hands straight above you, as far as you can, and let your palms and fingers relax.

Using your mind, direct all of your attention into the palms of your hands and your fingers. You have the ability to feel the vibrations of your environment in your hands and fingers. Think of them as antennae that allow you to "feel" sounds.

Imagine that your hands and fingers are starting to tune in to all of the sounds and vibrations around you—people talking, rush-hour traffic, the sounds of nature, anything. As this happens, your hands and fingers may want to move or just be still; let them do what they want. They will automatically filter out unpleasant sounds and vibrations that might cause you to feel upset or uneasy, leaving only instructive, uplifting, and positive experiences.

As you listen with your hands and fingers it is like playing a gigantic harp in your mind.

Use the sounds and vibrations to heal you, ease you, and develop vitality. Try to do this exercise two times a day for ten minutes each time.

CHAPTER TEN

Love, Laughter, and Dying

O ne evening when my soul was newly made, my teacher and I sat looking out across a lake in a mountain range on the North Island of New Zealand. We gazed at a mountain, at an arc of shooting stars, at the moon shy behind wispy clouds. I asked my teacher, "What should I learn now?"

"You must know how to die and come back to life again." He chuckled loudly. "Death is everywhere, mixed with life. Feel it, understand it."

I looked at the mountain across the valley. I felt it look back at me. It welcomed me, unfolding like a flower. I sent my soul into it and I learned of its birth in the time when time did not matter, of the land from which it rose, and of the plants and animals upon it, and I felt young, small, and at the start of the human species.

Running through these perceptions of the soul, like veins of gravity, was death. When I looked into death I saw that it was not a dark void but a brilliant black diamond. Within it was the gateway to liberation, in this life and all others.

I looked back to the mountain. "Mountains are libraries," murmured Ürgyen. I could sense that this mountain held the wisdom of the earth, and I had learned that the knowledge of death and the knowledge of the earth were connected.

I questioned my teacher again: "What should I have? What should I be?" A few minutes passed. He leaned toward me and whispered, "The power of a Ngagpa, the essence of a child, the wisdom of a philosopher, the healing of a mother, and the personality of a mountain."

The Gifts of Death

Many people in the West believe that no one can talk about death with any real insight because no one who has died has really come back to fill in the details. Tibetan wisdom, however, states very clearly that all of us have returned from the dead. Birth is only one half of death, according to the Tibetans, with life squeezed in between the two.

At the moment of death we are initiated into the great mystery of ourselves—the light of liberation. If we can hold on to the moment when we have the chance to be in this light and ascend into the height of this experience, then understanding of self, life, and death is ours.

We should start to think of death in all its aspects as part of our life experience. This does not mean you need to visit a cemetery regularly or keep the bones of your best friend under your bed; rather, contemplating death enables you to look into the most profound aspects of your consciousness, where life and death live together.

Living and dying are the same experience. Within ourselves and our lives, within our experience of death and possible rebirth, are varying states of consciousness: waking consciousness, dream consciousness, meditative consciousness, death-process consciousness, and the consciousness of reality and rebirth. We experience all of these states every day and every night in everything we do, from brushing our teeth in the morning to dreaming at night. As we die, our sensitivities become heightened and these states of consciousness become more transparent, allowing us to see them clearly. In the West we talk about the whole of a dying person's life flashing before him before facing judgment. Tibetan wisdom believes that those who are dying re-experience their lives, intensely and rapidly, both the good and the bad. The goal of this is that we gain self-knowledge and redeem ourselves, entering into a state of balance and peace. The danger is that we may be overwhelmed by these extremes of emotion. That is why the Tibetans place such importance on looking after the dying.

Another important thought to hold on to when looking at death is that the force of the universe is the same force as the human mind. The universe and the mind are constructed in the same way. In the process of dying and attaining spiritual liberation, the person is encouraged to hear with his or her intuition universal truths as well as personal ones. You become able to grasp reality—that profound and intimate moment in which you truly discover your innocence and inner knowledge—in a spontaneous way. I hope that in a similarly spontaneous way, you will be able to experience a connection with the ancient Tibetan wisdom of death and the art of dying.

Many people are afraid of death, but if we can come to associate ourselves with eternal energy, we lose the fear of death. At any important times in our lives, including the time of dying and death, we are brought closer to experiences of spiritual potential. This is specifically true as we die. During this in-between state, the dying person has access to opportunities for spiritual rejuvenation. Some of the experiences can be very frightening, because of their intensity, while others are comforting. Beneath them all, though, exists the essential energy and light of reality.

In death as in life, people can become confused, so Tibetan culture evolved ways to help people through this challenging time. It is challenging not only for the dying person but for those who are left behind. According to ancient teachings on death and dying, the dying person becomes highly vulnerable to the powerful emotions of those who are grieving his or her loss, and this can result in intense pain. Both in Buddhist and Bön teachings, there are texts and oral teachings designed to guide everyone involved in the dying process to a better state of mind. Normally a spiritual teacher reads the texts; in the absence of one, a sincere friend guides his dying comrade to happiness.

Spiritual teachers within the Tibetan traditions usually know all the guides to dying by heart. Many are in the form of prayers dedicated to compassionate deities that come to aid people through the scary moments of dying and into the beauty, fulfillment, and self-knowledge that intersperse them. The most important thing that Western readers can learn from this view of death and dying is that whatever we have done and whatever we have believed or not believed, we can transform our lives as we go through the different stages of dying.

My teacher was often asked to guide dying people who were not Tibetan but who wanted a way of bringing their lives to integrated conclusions. Once he was asked to help someone who lived far away. He invoked the consciousness of the person by making a picture of him on a clean white piece of paper. This ritual image, or *jangbu,* was laid on an altar. Then my teacher talked to the image of the dying person, explaining all the possible experiences to come, including the different realms of existence and their qualities.

After that, he took the drawing between his middle and

index fingers and held it over a small flame. As the fire consumed the image, he announced that all the unskillful actions and thoughts of this person had been cleared and purified. Tibetan wisdom believes that in the flames, the reformed consciousness of the subject finds its journey to a more fruitful life than the one it has just left.

Just as my teacher had finished this ritual, his telephone rang. It was the family of the dying person. As he had died, a radiant light had emanated from him, they told my teacher. The room had filled with many colored lights and sweet smells and the assembled family members and friends had experienced profound joy and calm.

A NEAR-DEATH EXPERIENCE

Some people who have died return to the world and tell others of their experiences. My teacher told me this story about Latri Gyalwa, a real Tibetan person, who had been studying how to build a soul when he had this experience.

Latri Gyalwa lost all his vitality to an incurable illness that came out of the blue. He began to die and as he started to cross from this world into the in-between state, he began to apply the little he could remember about creating a soul. For many days, he felt blown about like a flower on a strong wind. Then suddenly a guide appeared: a resplendent and radiant female being, whose appearance changed constantly from Jamma the Loving Mother to a mysterious woman whose face he could not see.

On their journey, he met many people who taught him about the nature of birth and death. He learned to respect all living creatures, to be a good person, and to value spiritual insight and spiritual teachers in whatever form or circumstances they might appear. After what seemed an endless time, he briefly encountered various lords of the dead. But much to the shock and amazement of everyone gathered around his deathbed, he returned to his body to tell them about what he had learned.

Not every person who had these near-death experiences in Tibet had them validated as real by their teachers. If they did—as with Latri—the people were known as "de-loks." The near-death experiences of the de-loks, which have been remembered or written down, are very similar to those of people who have had near-death experiences in the West.

Now let us go further into two important aspects of death: how to prepare for death—which also helps you prepare for living—and how to help the dying to die well, a crucial skill that can help to heal everyone and overcome all prejudices. These two aspects of the death process are embodied in the following five points of understanding. Consider them well. It is essential to accept and reflect on these points in order to benefit from Tibetan wisdom about death and dying.

The five points of understanding death and dying:

- Understand in your own terms what death is.

- Understand that it is important to be aware of this.

- Understand techniques for preparing for death.

- Understand the stages of the death experience.

- Understand the help that people need as they die.

Over the following pages we will explore the Tibetan view of death and your feelings about death. We will contemplate the nine ways of death and learn how to create happiness and die peacefully, with self-knowledge and empowerment.

The Tibetan View of Death

Life is transitory, so we must learn how to live our time carefully and with discretion. Tibetan spiritual practices of all traditions teach that awareness and meditation on death are vital in developing our consciousness. By understanding the death experience, we lose our fear of it and can start to transform all the other turbulent emotional processes that will come to the surface at the time of our death and dying.

Death and dying are two different experiences. Dying in calmness and mental clarity ensures calmness and clarity for those who mourn you and guides us to a better rebirth. Death is viewed as a permanent split of mind and body by the Tibetans. Our minds continue after our bodies have died and then take a new body as best they can.

All of us have had countless numbers of lives with little or no control over what type of lives they are. As we learn to gain control of this process, we can begin to become more self-determining. All our thoughts and actions, speech and deeds, written words and aspirations from previous lives leave their mark on our minds, like old layers of French polish on a piece of old furniture. These marks can be good, bad, or in between, depending on our actions (karma means "to act").

As we clean off each layer, we can gain insight about our karma. Remember, though, that while it is important to consider the legacy of karma from previous lives, it is far more important to concern ourselves with our karma in this life, as I explained in chapter 3.

Your Feelings About Death

Your individual state of mind is very important as you die. It influences how you will cope with the experience of dying and how you will be born into a new form of existence. By contemplating death, you can start to treat your life more sacredly, which will bring you peace of mind and a greater connection to reality.

In order to help ensure that you have a good death, you must try to work on yourself while you are living. Stop and think seriously about how you view death. You may think you have no thoughts or opinions about it at all, but deep within, you are bound to have feelings about it. All these feelings can help you to understand death. The emotions that attach themselves to death, both your own and others', usually include fear, loneliness, and anger. A sense of powerlessness is also a common experience. These emotions often seem crushing, but remember that dying people also feel a sense of peace, acceptance, spiritual joy, forgiveness, and total release from hardship and pain.

Anger is the biggest emotion that causes suffering of intense proportions for dying people, often causing them to be reborn in a less desirable life than they really deserve. Transforming negative states of mind is the hardest work we face—it is easier to conquer another country than to start releasing the negativity within.

Consider also that reality, as we experience it, is created by patterns made primarily of random thoughts that collide with one another, causing massive amounts of energy to be released, which give form and substance to our lives. These random thoughts could be anything from "I must pick up the laundry" or "What shall I have for dinner?" to "What is the meaning of life?" The process of dying and death reveals this random reality.

Many of us are uneasy about the whole idea of death and our culture tries in the main to ignore it. In fact, ever since the first human being realized that death was here to stay, there have been some basic reasons for why we feel so unsure about death. They are:

- Ego: We believe that each of us is an independent, self-existing personality, so how can this personality just stop? Suddenly we know that nothing lasts forever and this includes us. According to the Tibetan view, this is where all our troubles start.

- Lack of trust: Death creates so many uncertainties for us. Few of us know what goes on as we die, what happens after, or why we die, and we are reluctant to trust people who say they do know about it.

- Fear: We are often scared that death will be painful. We feel isolated by the idea of death and worried about those we leave behind.

All these notions seem valid. You probably know people who have gone through them or have experienced them yourself. But they do not really take place within our inner consciousness. They are fears that we have absorbed, since childhood, from other people. Peace of mind comes from recognizing that although they feel real to us, these fears are fantasy. Studying the nature of death helps us to know that we can be the authors of our deaths as well as our lives.

Contemplating the Nine Ways of Death

There is a direct relationship between our fears of living and our fears of death. Many people are afraid of life and its uncertainties because they feel that life is more powerful than they are. They are like this because they do not know how to change their inner state. The majority of dying people experience the same mental confusion. So it is important to have in place simple structures to remind us of basic truths.

The nine ways of death can do this for us. Reflect on them as often as you can. These nine ways of death are common to both Buddhism and Bön and are known by slightly different names in various spiritual traditions of Tibet. The nine ways are broken into three main areas of discussion.

We all are going to die:

1. Each one of us is dying right now, but in very tiny segments.

2. According to Tibetan wisdom, our life span is getting shorter in this particular stage of the world's time cycle, due to the spiritual pressures of overpopulation.

3. We treat death as if it happens only to other people.

Death comes without warning for many people:

4. No one knows when he or she will die.

5. Our physical bodies are not indestructible and do not live forever, no matter how we look after them.

6. Dying is a natural process and there are as many ways of dying as there are people.

Spiritual practice helps us at the point of death:

7. Spiritual practice will help us to die well and gain inner happiness; it doesn't matter what it is or whether or not we understand it.

8. Nothing we own, have worked for, or achieved can guide us through the dying experience; our physical bodies cannot assist us, their time has ended.

9. Our loved ones cannot come with us or make death easier. They can only wave good-bye. Equally, however, your enemies cannot harm you, as animosity will be left behind.

CONSIDER HOW THE BODY STOPS WORKING JUST BEFORE DEATH

Within Tibetan medicine and spiritual teachings are many techniques used for understanding the death process and all the signs of death. You can start to familiarize yourself with this process by thinking about how the body of a dying person slowly stops working as he grows near to death. Imagine what that looks and feels like; if you have spent time with a person in the process of dying, think back to that experience. Relate the process to your life as it is now. Being near dying people can be helpful, so you might consider working as a volunteer in a hospice.

HOW TO HELP OTHER PEOPLE WHO ARE ABOUT TO DIE

We can help others by first helping ourselves. Let us look at the following steps, which reflect everything we have learned in this book.

- Try to develop an acceptance of death. Do not be afraid of the process. As you understand more about death, so your fear will lose its sting.

- Try to live as best you can and be as good as you can. In particular, avoid killing, stealing, greed, anger, lust, aggression, using inappropriate sexual energy, or inappropriate and unskillful speech and language. These actions can cause death to be unpleasant because they create immediate psychic side-effects and diminish your vital energy.

- Find a way to understand your mind through a spiritual, religious, or ethical practice. Try to develop love for yourself and compassion for all living creatures. Find a practice that feels right for you, and then work hard to apply it. Whatever you do will help you if you are sincere. Following a spiritual practice puts death into its true perspective as another part of your cycle of life. My teacher taught me a contemplation practice that gave me insight about my life, my death, and my self. This exercise is called The Five Benefits of Developing Intention. It is a powerful self-healing exercise that creates immediate and long-term benefits in all parts of your life. It activates a powerful compassion that can eventually liberate you from your mental restrictions.

- Focus on whatever spiritual belief you have and see it purifying you—your speech, actions, thoughts, mind, and body. Then see it blessing the world around you.

- Create within your mind powerful and positive mental statements that negativity will not damage your inner life, that compassion is always within you, and that you are always trying to be compassionate.

- Look at the effects that negative emotions have on you and on other people. Consider how you create these emotions, how you attract them, and how they cause you damage.

- Pray never to be separated from the compassion and kindness that exists within you. Pray that other people may also find and keep this compassion and kindness.

- Reflect on how you suffer and why, think of all your hardships, then move on to consider how you can use the experiences to understand yourself more.

Death is our greatest teacher if we just know how to listen to what is being taught. It is important to start as early as possible. In order to understand death and what it has to offer, you must first look at your life. Do this by dividing your life into three sections:

- From birth to 20

- From 21 to 40

- From 41 up

If you are under 20, divide your age into three again, from birth to 10, from 10 to 15, and from 15 to 20. If you are in the 21 to 40 group, take the first category, then divide it again from 21 to 30, 30 to 35, or 35 to 40.

Next, write down one statement that is the essence of each age group. This has to do with your feelings, not what you achieved or did, but the underlying emotional reality for you at each stage of your life. You can identify the underlying essence of your life through the following meditation, which will show you both the nature of your past and how your life has progressed.

Sit quietly. Start with your current cycle. At first, don't focus on a particular thing or aspect, just let yourself float;

slowly, key elements will start to arise. Be gentle and quiet with yourself. You will start to identify the underlying theme. As you do so, direct your breath at it, and as your breath passes through, imagine that you are extracting its essence and purifying it of obstructions.

When you are at the second stage, direct to it as much kindness as you can. It then reveals itself. Repeat this with the third stage. Now you can start to reflect on the themes and learn from them. Rest in this last stage, considering what you have found out and its relevance to your life.

This simple practice will bring great insight. Not only will happiness increase and problems decrease, but fear and other mental impressions will become less intense or will disappear. By doing this meditation regularly, you will create a deep inner peace.

When you come to the time for death, this peace will be with you, you will know why you had to die, and there will be no fear. On the day you decide to die physically, your inner mental world will become illuminated with the clear light of love and consciousness. You will wake up to a new horizon, and your self-created soul—a fusion of intellect and will, imagination and symbolic understanding—will navigate a small but indestructible boat that will guide you across a great ocean to your ultimate destination.

Giving Love and Kindness to a Dying Person

Now let us look at simple and compassionate ways to help people who are about to die. Giving love and kindness to a dying person is a miraculous act that anyone can do. But often our own fears, prejudices, attachments, and ambitions get in the way.

Think instead of all the good experiences you have had in your life. They were created by good energy. You can direct that same powerful vitality to help the dying person go on their way with greater ease and mental clarity.

Everyone's death is meaningful. Sometimes, though, neither they nor those left behind discover the meaning. By following some of the suggestions below, you may help the dying person discover the meaning of his life, and you may discover the meaning of yours.

Honesty, understanding, the desire for freedom, respect, love, and acceptance are key in creating a beneficial relationship between the person who is dying and those who are caring. Honesty is important; in this context it means that you should always be yourself, that the way you are inside is important. Give as best as you are able. Your heart is wisdom; it knows what to listen for, if you let it. Be straightforward and sensitive when you express your feelings. Remember that at any time you could be in the dying person's place.

Understanding comes from your heart's perception of your interchanges with the dying person. Often it's not what you say that is important. Don't let your ego or his get in the way. Do not be a know-it-all. Be as empathetic as you can, for that is what the dying person needs.

The desire for freedom is often a struggle at this time, as the person clings to memories of life yet also wants to die and be at peace. Sometimes a dying person seeks assurance that he can die, that he is not being irresponsible by dying and leaving everyone else to pick up the pieces. Always assist if you can with unfinished domestic matters. This will help the person die with fewer attachments to this life and a calm sense from having put things in order.

Another aspect of freedom is that the dying person is able to look back and stop regretting the big events that he or she had formerly regarded as setbacks or bad situations. When people die with regrets, they are slowed down on the path to happiness, and the regrets linger in the minds of those who are left behind.

Always respect the goodness in people. Respect is crucial to a dying person's feeling safe and secure, just as it is for those of us who are living. No one has a right to judge a dying person. Individuals are their own judge, jury, and redeemer. Remind them that they are brave and that their example brings hope to other people.

Dying people feel love intensely when it is directed toward them. Love creates an immediate connection that reassures the dying person that he is protected. The very experience gives them hope. Acceptance is crucial in caring for dying people. One day they will be happy and the next they will be gloomy. Many pent-up emotions can also explode at this time. Don't be offended by what they say. Ignore their words but not their being.

Practically speaking, the best thing anyone can do for a dying person is to make things as uncomplicated as possible, from the physical environment to the visits of friends and family.

Try not to become attached to dying people because this will act like a psychic glue to them after they are dead. They will want to be with you, and not move on. Listen carefully to whatever a dying person says, for his words are statements of his being, but do not enter into powerful or intense emotional encounters.

It is very helpful to empower a dying person by encouraging him to use whatever spiritual beliefs he has to focus his consciousness. In the room where he is, place some type of uplifting picture, or a statue or image that represents his belief. Have it close to the person in case he wishes to touch it. If the dying person has no structured beliefs or is an atheist, help him, or her, to discover beauty in himself and in other people. Helping dying people to focus on peace and positive examples of life and beauty enables them to experience those qualities. As they do this, any fear, anger, or other powerful emotion will lose some of its bite.

If you have known the dying person well for a long time, you may see a completely different dimension to this person's character and personality. If so, don't force on him anything such as a religious practice—confession, for instance—or mind-altering drugs, with the misguided belief that it is good for him. It could cause the person serious emotional injury—and you as well.

The most important aspect of care for dying people is to honor their mental integrity. Encourage them to dwell on freedom and inspire them to hold thoughts of compassion and happiness in their minds as much as possible. If the dying person dies thinking of the well-being of others, then that will happen. Focusing on taking the burden of another's suffering, and returning compassion to others, creates a huge resource of positive energy and love. It will also help the person to die with a heightened state of consciousness.

As much as you are able, try to understand the mental patterns of the dying person's mind. If the individual is open, discuss with him how he has seen his life. If someone is unconscious, you can communicate with her as if she were awake and listening to you. Direct positive thoughts to these people; think of the energy permeating through their unconsciousness into their inner selves and transmitting all your good wishes, warm intentions, and compassion.

If someone is in physical pain, it is good to use medications to eliminate this pain. If people are in mental pain, however, it is not good to sedate them because they will die even more confused than they were before they started to die. You can give them positive help by directing emotional calm and love to them, and by improving the colors and ambience of their immediate surroundings, with flowers, for instance.

Dying people are very sensitive to their immediate environment and to the mental energies of other people. Family disharmony and other arguments can cause profound emotional pain for the dying person. So peace should be made between everyone.

Finally, don't neglect the lighter side. Dying people love to be entertained, so find out what form of art or entertainment they like the most and let them have as much as they want. It acts as a mental food, filling them up with positive energy.

Blessing for the Dead

This mixture of a prayer, benediction, and creation of vital energy is uplifting and profound for those who are left behind. It is designed to help the dead and heal the bereaved.

> *Good Friend, you have died,*
> *soon you are about*
> *to leave your body never to return.*
> *Your actions here are finished,*
> *You can take nothing with you on your way.*
> *All regrets, troubles, and pain*
> *now no longer have a claim upon you.*
> *Let your face receive the Clear Light.*
> *You are pure now, no blemish or stain.*
> *Hold on to your highest belief.*
> *It anchors you like a kite in the strong wind.*
> *Become unified with the divine.*
> *Let your spiritual friends guide you to unity.*
> *Good Friend, give blessings to all things.*
> *Compassion is with you on your way.*

As you say this, direct a sphere of brilliant white light to the top of the dying or dead person's head. Think of it flowing down through him, purifying his body and consciousness, into his physical heart. Then direct the light up to the crown and out into the person's field of consciousness.

Do this as soon as the person is dead and each day for forty-nine days, as the dead person travels through the complex stages of coming to terms with dying. Another thing you can do for the dead person in this period is to be as gentle and compassionate to others as possible and, on the dead person's behalf, study any spiritual belief he or she may have had. This helps them and it helps you.

Always try to have funeral rites, undertakers, or whatever else planned beforehand. It makes life easier for you and the dead person. Let there be peace around them and at their funeral. The dead will be curious about how others see them, so they will want to be there, but loud noises at funerals can shock people who have recently died and cause them to panic because they have not fully come to terms with being dead.

After a Death

Whether you are a professional care-giver, a family member, or a close friend, you will be fragmented after someone dies, even if you don't feel you are. Life is never the same again. Once you have time to reflect, you will probably feel a mixture of emotions: worn out and anxious, relieved and angry, sad and happy. You may feel that life is a mixture of fantasy and reality. You might want to spend time alone, then suddenly need to be with people (always do both).

Everyone grieves in his or her own fashion. Share your feelings with a friend or friends and/or with a professional therapist. Crying can be helpful, but cry for yourself rather than cling to the dead person. If there was any unfinished business between you, give it up, douse it with love, and let it go. You are unable to change the past. If we hold on to memories of the dead person with too much force, we will create intense pain for ourselves and for others, because pain is contagious and can be spread in the emotional atmosphere.

This gentle prayer helps with pain and loss. It invokes healing and directs changes within yourself. My teacher called this particular prayer a Zor—or bomb—of happiness. In Bön, symbolic bombs were used to create transformative experiences in times of death or if there were obstructions in people's lives that could not be moved in any way. You may think that taking on the world's suffering is the last thing you want to do, but if you can be this selfless, the benefits are immeasurable. Say the entire prayer aloud, quietly, addressing it to all human beings and other living creatures.

All the world knows pain and grief,
All living creatures know this to be true.
All living creatures want to be free from suffering
And for pain never to return.
I do.
In this moment I am suffering.
I dedicate my suffering to all Life.
I take all the suffering of other living creatures
Upon me now, in order
That they may be free from grief and affliction.
May all pain of loss and unkindness be vanquished,
All our cruelty shall no longer prowl
as a blood-lusting tiger
within us now.
Let all suffering come to an end.
I cast this prayer into the world
And with my pure incoming breath destroy the
Dross and violence of this time
And blackness comes into my heart,
There my pain and loss die
Transformed from out of darkness into the healing brilliance

Of the clear light,
And as my breath rushes out in power, compassion, and
*   beauty*
All beings are free from suffering!

When My Teacher Died

A small clay bowl was placed in my hands. It was tied by a white silk scarf that fluttered in the evening wind. It held some of Ürgyen's ashes. His family gave them to me. It was what he wanted, they said.

I was not sad at my teacher's death, for sadness had no place. My teacher had come to an end in this life, but what he was continued on in others and myself. He died well, his mind in good health and his body tired.

I took his ashes back to Mount Pihanga and built a mound of rocks in which I lit a fire. I offered up prayers and blessings to my teacher, his family and his teachers, and the world at large. I placed the small clay bowl into the heart of the fire. It began to melt, encapsulating the ashes. I let the fire burn down, and as the melted bowl cooled, it formed a black sphere of concentrated spiritual power and blessing.

Taking the sphere to the edge of Lake Rotoponamu, which lies at the edge of Mount Pihanga, I threw the sphere far out into the lake. Finding the deepest part, it sunk to merge its energy with the water, fire, earth, wind, and sky of the volcanic land, there to radiate blessings and strong energy to all living beings. To this very day, the blessing sphere lies within the lake.

I returned to the little shrine of rocks, the fire still smoldering within it. Prayer flags fluttered gently in the evening wind. A purple sky stretched around me and out to the horizon. My teacher's flat drum hummed as the wind ran across its surface.

I stared off into the valley below, wondering what I was to do with all that I had learned.

Even though my teacher had encouraged me to find a way to bring these teachings to a Western understanding, I still felt uncertain. Then words that Ürgyen had spoken years before came back to me. "There is no need to doubt, just be at peace and the answers will come."

I threw more wood into the fire. "Look for the answers, then you'll know the questions."

The smell of rain floated on the breeze. "Nothing is as it seems." My teacher's voice was faint, distant. I looked up and saw a cascade of shooting stars.

Postscript

Every aspect or experience of our lives, each memory, fear, success, dream, or aspiration, is a gift that holds within it the magic of health, happiness, and sacredness.

True health has nothing to do with doctors or healers of any type. It has to do with inner purity, power, and patience. This comes by understanding the value in our suffering. It means that we have to work hard as we go through the processes of physical, psychological, and spiritual change.

This is the hardest thing that any person can do and you can only do it on your own. Of course, there are others who can help, but ultimately it's up to you.

As you heal yourself you will begin to find insight into the nature of knowledge and the love that exists in all of humanity. Every person is sacred. Every person is Love encapsulated into a special form and personality. Knowing this even a little connects each of us to happiness because happiness is a taste of the sacred in all things.

Simply by the act of starting to heal your life, you spark the healing of others and of the world in which we live. You don't need to force this idea on other people. The quiet act of living in accordance with who you are and who you can be allows the natural influence of goodness to grow.

As this goodness finds its own expression in other people there comes with it wisdom and knowledge—knowledge of the natural world and of the inner workings of human nature, of the power of mind and thought in the material world. Ngagpas were the first beings of the ancient world to have this knowledge. They passed it on not just to their descendants but into the psyche—the spiritual core—of all humanity.

Humanity at large, which includes all of us, has been sick for a very long time. We have forgotten our intrinsic nature. We have lost sight of the knowledge that along with our instinct for survival are the instincts of spiritual wisdom, healing, and happiness. When we forget that we have these qualities of inner wisdom we become unhappy. Unhappiness makes us sick. And so the cycle continues.

All we have to remember is that we, all of us, are the cure.

As you start to understand your mind and the nature and limitations of your thought, you will—sooner or later—come to a place of consciousness that is vast and out of your normal experience. Our normal experiences are dependent on our everyday minds. The everyday mind believes that it has an everyday consciousness so it becomes shy, doubtful, and needy, and feels impotent. Exposed to the raw pain of this, many people do not have lives at all: Life is an iceberg and they are underwater. Others build apparently successful lives because they contrive to stay on top of the iceberg by dint of paying no attention to the fact that they will slowly melt into this vast consciousness and disappear.

Yet, in this everyday self is an essence of higher consciousness that is uniquely who you are. It pervades all things, from sea to sky, from the first to be born and the last to die, and you are in communion with all things. Every day becomes one day, a day of gladness and beauty that reinvents itself as you do through the natural delight of creation.

How is this achieved? By developing the ability of balance. This is not the weighing of one thing against the other, or the unskillful action of running from one action to the next, but knowing that true balance comes out only in the spaces between moments. You must believe not in time but in the effects of time.

In order to know balance, we must know our history. This is not just the passing of events—personal, social, cultural, and global—but the engraving of our consciousness upon our selves. As a species, our biggest injustice to one another and to ourselves—beyond cruelty, war, and disease—is that we forget our interconnectedness with all other living creatures. We pull ourselves back into the everyday mind and believe we are separate from others, above, below, different, and therefore not responsible.

We are not separate. We are all the face of whatever God we believe in. Although we are all born and die with inequalities, we must strive to attain a common equality that lies not in external achievements but in the spirituality, the unity, and the beauty of our humanity.

We are love, wisdom, and compassion. We are our greatest achievement and our greatest degradation. We are mystery and clarity. We are the great laughter that we can hear when we listen closely to the workings of the universe in nature and in our hearts. We are the universe, the cosmos rising up to recognize us. We are the cosmos in descent, bringing down spiritual wisdom to be used in the world of time and the everyday mind.

From infancy, all of us search for an animating principle or experience in our lives. We do this through stories, beliefs, and events that are redolent of significance and value. Things beyond our imagination somehow support this principle, allowing us to transcend our everyday minds. This is the interface where impossible things can be actual and meaningful, where wonder and faith intermingle. Where all things are acknowledged.

Many people consider faith crazy and ridiculous, but it is exactly this: When we have faith, we can move beyond the set beliefs of our society into the absolute freedom of pure consciousness.

The starting place is to go back to the outlook we had as children. Most of us know that young children believe in everything and it is in this mind-set that we can develop discernment and consciousness and discover faith.

The first step to faith is the belief in all things; the second is the experience that Everything believes in each of us. This exists within us now. We know this, yet we are afraid. We have this ready to experience, yet we shy away. Opening the door to it is our gift to ourselves.

That is the Tibetan art of living.

Consulting a Physician of Tibetan Medicine

If you wish to consult a physician of Tibetan medicine, I urge you to make sure that whoever you see is qualified and competent. At the time of writing this, there is no register of physicians of Tibetan medicine, either Buddhist or Bön, but an international association is being established.

The first consultation may last from ten minutes to two hours, depending on how the physician views your condition and what is best suited to your needs. Subsequent appointments may take place at weekly, monthly, or three-month intervals. The cost is likely to range from £10 to £100 ($14.50 to $150.00), or a donation, depending on the needs of the physician.

Here are a few simple guidelines to help you get the most from the initial consultation and subsequent treatments.

Ask direct questions and expect clear answers: Don't be afraid to ask questions and to go on asking them until you receive clear answers that you understand fully.

Diagnosis: The "absolute treatment" is in fact the diagnosis, according to Tibetan medicine. True and accurate diagnosis gives a physician insight into how your mental, emotional, and physical systems interact. This insight should activate your self-healing potential and help you to feel peaceful and clear. Usually, the physician will also tell you the prognosis if you do not make the recommended changes to your life-style in terms of food, diet, behavior, and so on.

The three main techniques of diagnosis:

- The physician examines the patient for symptoms and indications that can be observed in appearance, character, personality, and speech; the physician also studies the urine and other bodily excretions and the eyes and tongue. Take a sample of urine (150–200 ml/5–7 fl. oz.) to the first consultation.

- Touching the patient with respect and sensitivity, the physician studies pulse, temperature, body growth patterns, skin, bones, and finger- and toenails, and closely inspects troubled areas of the body. Pulse diagnosis will reveal the nature and types of illness in the patient. From this, an experienced physician can determine how the complaint first came into being and the best form of treatment. This will help you to understand not only what is wrong but why, and how you can heal both your illness and your life. If possible, try to be relaxed when you see the physician, as this can help in carrying out an accurate pulse diagnosis; if you have any spiritual practice or belief, focus on it before seeing the physician. However, a good physician can help regardless of your spiritual state.

- The physician takes a medical history including dietary and behavioral habits, symptoms, illnesses, and diseases, and the effects of season and climate changes.

Medication: Most traditional Tibetan medicines can safely be taken with Western pharmacological drugs, but make sure that your Tibetan doctor knows and understands any drugs you are taking, because this may affect what they prescribe.

Life-style changes: Physicians should be able to deal with all types of influences on your health that affect you at the time of consultation. Life-style changes are key to treatment, but they may recommend changes that you are unable or unwilling to make. If this happens, do not be afraid to discuss these and negotiate. If you can, however, and if you trust the physician, it is preferable to carry out his or her advice.

Further Information

If you would like to know more about Christopher Hansard's work, and that of the other practitioners at the Eden Medical Centre, please contact:

Sharon Seager
Communications Manager
Eden Medical Centre
63a King's Road
London SW3 4NT
Telephone: 011-44-20 7881 5800

E-mail: SAS@edenmedicalcentre.com
Website: www.edenmedicalcentre.com

Index